Wave Goodbye to Type 2 Diabetes

Published by *Holistic Remedy Publishing*
Cover Design: *Fresh Design* at https://mfairbanks.carbonmade.com/
Editing and Formatting: D.J. Natelson
ISBN: 978-0-578-41929-9

WAVE GOODBYE TO
TYPE 2 DIABETES

16 Holistic Practices to
Prevent & Reverse Diabetes
& Reclaim Joy, Vitality, & Plenty

NICKI STEINBERGER, PH.D.

DISCLAIMER

The content in this book is meant for informational and educational purposes only. Dr. Nicki's teachings and the *Holistic Practices Lifestyle* (*HPL*) are not meant to diagnose, treat, or cure any disease. The *HPL* is not a substitute for consultations with your health care practitioner or medical advisor. Readers should seek guidance from their licensed health practitioner before making changes to their medications, and before adopting new dietary or exercise regimes. The information provided here can be helpful to the management of type 2 diabetes in many cases, but individuals vary in their medical condition and needs, so consultation with a personal health care provider is mandatory. Whatever information or recommended products you choose to use, you are self-prescribing. As such, Dr. Nicki and the *HPL* assume no responsibility.

Thank you for your mindfulness,
Dr. Nicki

CONTENTS

RESOURCES

Resources Page: To provide added value and support, I have created supplemental guides. These guides will both deepen your focus in particular areas and give you easy-to-follow blueprints. They're available on my resources page* and include:

- ✓ 10 Top Foods to Stock Your Kitchen for Optimal Health
- ✓ 7 Nutritional Supplements to Reverse Type 2 Diabetes
- ✓ 10 Holistic Lifestyle Practices to Prevent & Reverse Disease (beginning and advanced)
- ✓ 5 Medicinal Green Juice Recipes & Easy Start Guide (eBook)

Private Facebook Group: I coined the phrase: "Life-Power, not willpower!" This means focusing on expansion and growth rather than contraction and restriction. Mindset shifts like this have an extraordinary way of producing desired results. This is how we roll and what we seek to cultivate in the Joy, Vitality, & Plenty Community.[†] I would love to have you join us.

Your Review of the Book: To spread the word on the healing potential of a holistic practices, and help folks determine if this book is the right fit for them, I would greatly appreciate your honest review on Amazon.[‡]

---

* http://drnickisteinberger.com/waveresources/
† http://drnickisteinberger.com/community
‡ http://drnickisteinberger.com/wavereview

PART ONE:
WE BEGIN

THE YEAR I REVERSED TYPE 2 DIABETES

Before I tell you my story, let's start with a definition of type 2 diabetes. In simple terms, type 2 diabetes (diabetes mellitus) is a metabolic condition. It is the inability of your body to use the hormone insulin effectively. Produced by the pancreas, insulin is necessary for transporting glucose (sugar) from your bloodstream to your individualized cells.

This process gives you the vital, daily energy you need to function properly. When your cells are not receptive and do not allow glucose to enter, a condition known as insulin resistance occurs. When enough glucose is not removed from your bloodstream, your blood glucose levels increase. Over time, this can lead to a diabetic condition.

***

In March 2010, at age 45, I was diagnosed with type 2 diabetes. I didn't want to face the symptoms I was experiencing—tremor-like shaking, incredible fatigue that left me crashed out in the afternoon, increased thirst, frequent urination, extreme mood swings, chronic yeast infections, and rashes on both sides of my body.

I was unsteady, having trouble focusing … and two years deep into a doctoral dissertation in clinical psychology. I needed help fast. In fact, I needed a radical transformation.

A family member strongly suggested I get tested for type 2 diabetes. She knew the symptoms—had experienced them with someone close to her—and recognized them in me. I resisted getting tested for a couple of years. While I denied the undeclared diagnosis, secretly, I worried it might be true.

Years before—it must have been 1997—I'd had a psychic reading from a well-regarded woman in the community where I lived. Her name was June. She had long, dark hair and a big Los Angeles smile. In her spacious Malibu Canyon apartment, I sat elevated on a platform with a large white wall behind me. She stood a few yards in front of me and proceeded to "read the writing on the wall." She tuned in to the entities and ancients she felt in the room with us, and they gave her messages.

At the time, something she said stood out. She was trying to identify a message coming through to do with health and illness but was having trouble. She said, "No, it's not diabetes."

I wondered for the longest time why diabetes had even entered her vision. Now, I realized it was because she had been picking up on something that *was* there, or that was on its way. But I still didn't want to get tested.

In 2010, 13 years after my psychic reading with June, a hemoglobin A1C (HbA1c) test was ordered for me after my fasting blood glucose results came in at 132 mg/dL. (For reference, 100 milligrams per deciliter and over is cause for concern, although further testing is needed to determine a type 2 diabetes diagnosis.)

I clearly remember the day I sat down with my practitioner and she told me my HbA1c was 8.9%. Diagnosis confirmed.

My practitioner prescribed an oral diabetes medication called metformin. I left the office with the prescription in my hand, knowing very well I was not going to fill it anytime soon—if at all. I am not suggesting this for you, as it was a personal decision, and the right one for me at the time.

I had what I call *a healthy aversion to chemical pharmaceuti-*

cals. I did not believe they had the power to heal or help me. I also had a head start: I believed in the effectiveness of lifestyle medicine and had been studying and researching holistic health and natural living for many years.

Surprisingly, the diagnosis freed me—and came as a relief. It was a blessing, because I finally knew what I was dealing with and could therefore get to work treating it.

(So much for timing! It took me two more years to finish my half-done dissertation. Saying it *wasn't* an easy task is a huge understatement.)

I was done avoiding my diagnosis. It was time to dive in.

Diabetes is a condition, not a disease. It thrives in a particular environment and diminishes in another. I made it my mission to create a diminishing environment and reverse my type 2 diabetes naturally … holistically.

I researched everything on the topic I could find. I listened to and watched health educators, doctors, wise healers, and everyday people share what they knew about applying a holistic healing protocol to restore balance and create a healthy, thriving system. I felt inspired.

When I found a holistic diabetes recovery program in the Southwest, I was extremely excited. That is, until I noticed the price tag for the program was over $10,000. No way! No access for me. What was I going to do? I needed this. I discovered I knew the wife of the director of the program. Many years ago, she had been my first yoga teacher in Santa Cruz, CA, and we had had a great connection!

I considered writing her a letter asking if there were some way she could help me get into the program. Then I thought about all the other folks who did not have access, and I decided not to support a business that denied entry to so many everyday people. Disappointed, I let it go.

In my quest to take back my health, I could not find a treatment protocol or method that was right for me. This led me to mix and match. I chose the best of the best; integrated it with my own knowledge, research, and intuition; and created a holistic approach to reversing diabetes.

Going against the grain of the mainstream culture did not come without obstacles. Fear told me to question my decision to treat diabetes naturally. Family, friends, the Western medical establishment, film, TV, and advertising all said I must take pharmaceuticals, or I would end up with serious health complications. People close to me as well as the cultural mainstream voice around me echoed the same concern—that I was taking my life into my own hands. Only my partner and my brother (both of whom also believed in the power of holistic medicine to heal) supported me 100%. It took all my confidence and gumption to stand strong in my beliefs.

Thank goodness I did.

***

The next 12 months were an experiment with results unknown. I trusted the process, because I trusted the notion that healing would occur, and transformation was possible … if I practiced.

I practiced daily in areas of diabetes-specific nutrition, moving my body, veggie juicing, stress-reduction, tending to my sugar-flour addiction, and exercising my creative self-expression.

There were two main foods I cut from my meal plan. (That is, if you can call them food; they had little nutritional value.) The first was natural sodas—"natural" meaning "fruit-sweetened." I loved my natural sodas with a fierce grip and paired them with whatever I was eating. In fact, food without the soda was undeniably less appealing, and could even alter my mood to *disgruntled and frustrated*. If there was one thing I didn't want to share, it was my natural soda.

The second food I eliminated (or rather, cut down by 90%) was flour products. This included bread in its many shapes and forms, such as bagels, crackers, cookies, cake, pasta, and fried foods covered in flour. This was not easy. These were foods I lied for and hid in inconspicuous bags. I tucked myself into secret corners around town to indulge my addiction—consuming moist, fluffy, flour-sugar concoctions. I separated myself from those close to me, as though I were living a separate life. I was.

***

It's tempting to think that cutting certain foods or ingredients out of your meal plan is enough to transform your health. However, I learned that healthy eating isn't only about eliminating the bad; equally important is adding the good. This is what I call *getting the good stuff in.*

I took to the juice ... veggie juicing, that is. With the juicer firmly stationed on my kitchen counter and the good stuff on hand, making, drinking, and actually chewing green juice became a daily practice. Celery, cucumber, leafy greens (chard, spinach, kale, dandelion, romaine), and rotations of ginger, lemon, parsley, and cilantro—up to a quart of medicine daily went into my body, blood, and cells.

I took to the streets—or the sidewalks, anyway. With iPod in hand, headphones on ears, and in great anticipation and delight, I started walking loops around my neighborhood. You gotta love those Oakland, CA, hills ... and I did. The thing about hills is that you don't have to walk quickly to increase your heart rate and have an effective workout; the hills take care of that for you. I started with one or two loops up and down the hills; eight weeks in, I was looping five times. After 50 minutes and two podcasts, I felt like a new person. I was able to sustain this practice five to six days a week.

I also took the good advice of a holistic, organic chef who happened to be my partner, Chef Laur. Before it became the craze it is today, she told me I needed to increase my healthy fat intake as well as pay attention to my protein consumption. I was reluctant because I was not wise in this area of nutrition; I was predominantly focused on juicing and eating more raw plant foods.

Fortunately, she cooked for me too, and made sure I got the nutrition I needed. Her meals, as part of the food program she created, were a significant factor in helping me reverse diabetes. She made sure I consumed generous servings of coconut oil, extra virgin olive oil, raw nuts and seeds, and omega-3 fatty fish such as wild salmon and sardines. Her meals were art, and she could make them out of scraps if that's all I *thought* I had.

I am forever grateful to her. You can learn more about California Superfood Chef at californiasuperfoodchef.com.

***

Fast forward one year to March 2011.

Age 46. The tremor-like shaking had stopped. My mood had found even ground. The rashes on both sides of my body were gone. My chronic yeast infections had stopped.

What would the lab results show? Would the numbers reflect how well I was feeling? Had my diagnosis changed, matching the elimination of my symptoms?

My HbA1c came in at 6.3%, down from the previous 8.9%.

I was shocked. I couldn't believe it. I checked the name at the top of the lab results to make sure it was mine. My LDL cholesterol and triglycerides (fat in the blood) had also decreased significantly—over 100 points. I had lost over 40 pounds.

At that moment, I discovered my calling.

I would veer from psychotherapy into holistic health education. I would spread the word and help others take back their health naturally.

I created the *Holistic Practices Lifestyle (HPL)* to prevent and reverse type 2 diabetes and began teaching it to everyday people.

THE INSPIRATION

This is what happened: I began to hear the needs of the people in my communities.

While teaching small-group interactive workshops on preventing and reversing type 2 diabetes in the San Francisco Bay Area, California, and through my social media channels, I heard people around me start to speak up. Folks who received my email newsletters, read my blog posts and eBook on veggie juicing, and engaged with me via Facebook, Snapchat, Instagram, Pinterest, and Twitter, asked for what they needed. They said:

- I want to prevent or reverse type 2 diabetes.
- I need to make small changes, and it has to be simple.
- I'm afraid of being on medication forever.
- I'd rather not go on medication at all.
- I'm looking for a more natural way to go about this.
- What I've been doing hasn't been working.
- I feel overwhelmed with all the information.
- Can you help me?
- … and much more.

Wave Goodbye to Type 2 Diabetes is my response.

If you are new to my teachings, a big hello and welcome aboard! I am writing to you as a seeker on the paths of *simply wanting to feel better* and *being willing to take incremental, daily steps toward optimal health.*

It's my calling in this life to help us everyday people take back our health by breaking through the old myths and limiting beliefs about health and illness that have been injuring us for a long time. I'm a conduit for putting the power of good health back into the hands of the people, and my tools are holistic health education and daily practices.

In this book, I am going to teach you exactly what you need to know.

SYMPTOMS SPECTRUM

BEGIN WHERE YOU ARE!

You are a unique individual. Your next step toward optimal health will be determined by where you are right now in regard to your current lifestyle practices and your overall health on all levels—mentally, physically, emotionally, and spiritually.

YOU must begin where YOU are and take YOUR next step.

In regard to type 2 diabetes, I'm going to say it straight out: it's the number one risk factor for heart disease. There are many reasons for this, one of which is an increased level of low-grade inflammation in the arterial lining.[1] You'll be hearing a lot more about inflammation as you continue reading, because it has a huge impact on your health.

I don't mean to scare you, but time is of the essence for taking charge of your health and getting creative with your healing. Preventing and reversing diabetes can be approached with a fun, playful, and empowering attitude; there is just no time for excuses or procrastination.

We are all on the same continuum, somewhere in between *Chaos of Symptoms*, *Symptom Reduction/Elimination*, and *Optimal Health*.

CHAOS OF SYMPTOMS

By the time many of us are in our 20s and 30s, we find ourselves stuck in a *Chaos of Symptoms*. This is a place where we experience a range of subtle to debilitating symptoms and may have already been diagnosed with one or multiple health conditions. Symptoms may include, but are not limited to, poor digestion; lack of sleep; back, neck, or joint pain; depression; anxiety; high blood sugar; high blood pressure; headaches; fatigue; lack of energy; intense mood swings; negative side effects from chemical pharmaceuticals; and addictions.

SYMPTOM REDUCTION/ELIMINATION

As you take small, incremental, and consistent steps moving through the practices I outline below, you will gradually (or sometimes quickly) find your way to *Symptom Reduction/Elimination*. This is the place where you start to feel better. It seems miraculous, but it is not a miracle, per se; it is a result of your time, energy, effort, willingness, and mindset. Your aches, pains, and myriad of symptoms will lessen or disappear altogether. You will feel renewed with hope, a strong sense of comfort, and an increased sense of self.

Symptom Reduction/Elimination is a beautiful landing place that reflects your intentions and successes on the road to recovery. You might stop here, as many folks do; that is absolutely fine. You can give yourself the applause you rightfully deserve.

OPTIMAL HEALTH

There is another level of a quality of life that is yours if you desire. It is the place of *Optimal Health*. Here, you can live with a high level of joy, vitality, and plenty. This is the breeding ground for awakened consciousness and depth of purpose. This is holistic living at its best and supports the essence of who you are—body, mind, and spirit. You can heal fully when your entire self is integrated, nourished, and loved.

So what does this look like? *Optimal Health* is different for everyone, so you must define it for yourself. However, after working and speaking with many people, I have identified common qualities. Take to heart the ones that speak to you, and continue to recognize and identify your own.

In body: You feel rested and have energy when you need it. You are digesting well. Your vital signs are in range, and you are free from diagnoses. You feel little to no pain most of the time. You experience inner vitality. You sleep well. Your mood is steady. You are hormonally well-balanced. You feel magnificent.

In mind: You are able to live in the present moment. You think positively. You make healthy choices for yourself. You are able to choose your thoughts and responses. You feel a sense of calm.

In spirit: You see life's lessons and challenges as blessings. You practice self-love and self-forgiveness. You are at peace and grounded. You feel connected to yourself, others, and the Earth. You use your creative self-expression to give value to others and to yourself. You experience a strong sense of purpose. You see the loving essence in all those along your path.

ACID AND ALKALINE

Disease and *Chaos of Symptoms* tend not to live in an alkaline environment; they thrive in an acid-based culture. When your system is overly acidic, inflammation is on the rise. Inflammation in time can lead to imbalance and its negative effects—such as type 2 diabetes.

Consider this your opportunity to become an alchemist, learning to transform your body from an acidic to an alkaline environment. Optimally, you want to maintain an alkaline pH balance of 7.35–7.45.

You do not have to make multiple changes all at once. In fact, most people succeed when they make small, incremental, and sustainable adjustments. You are simply going to take YOUR next step at YOUR preferred pace.

What creates an acidic internal environment? Chemical pharmaceuticals, GMOs (genetically modified organisms), dangerous food-like products, processed foods, dairy products, animal-based foods, stress (do not take this lightly), many oils, most grains, some nuts, alcohol, tobacco, coffee, table salt, artificial sweeteners, and sugar.

What creates an alkaline internal environment? Plant-based foods; stress reduction; meditation; moving your body; veggie juicing; most vegetables; herbs; raw, living foods; most ripe fruit; some spices; and some nuts and seeds.[2]

Does this mean that you must only consume what is alkaline and never consume what is acidic? No, it doesn't. The idea here is to boost your awareness and knowledge in order to understand the choices you make and the effects they can and will have on your health.

The path to reversing and preventing type 2 diabetes (and other inflammation-related conditions) is to increase alkalizing foods and lifestyle choices while decreasing acidic foods and behaviors.

WEIGHT IS NOT THE BOTTOM LINE

Eighty to ninety percent of folks carrying type 2 diabetes also experience obesity.[3] You notice I say "experience" obesity because it is a condition, not a way to describe who you are. That leaves ten to twenty percent of diabetics not carrying excess weight. This is because weight is not the bottom-line cause of diabetes.[4]

Carrying more weight than is healthy for you is a symptom, just as metabolic syndrome, high blood sugar, and pre-diabetes are symptoms. Stop chastising yourself; let go of feeling guilty about your body shape, size, or eating behaviors. Right here, right now, the blame needs to shift.

The average American every year consumes 29 pounds of French fries, 23 pounds of pizza, 24 pounds of ice cream, 57 gallons of soda, 24 pounds of artificial sweeteners, 2.7 pounds of salt, 90,000 milligrams of caffeine, 152 pounds of sugar, 146 pounds of white flour, and 600 pounds of dairy.[5]

If you want to point a finger (though doing so is generally not effective), point it at the big food corporate industry. We are surrounded by gigantic pools of poison masked as food. Do you have to consume it? No, of course not. But when you are part of the masses being marketed to, perhaps since childhood, and cravings and addiction have set it, just saying "no" isn't easy. So take a step back and be gentle with yourself. You are not to blame.

The bottom line or root foundation of type 2 diabetes is insulin resistance.

Insulin resistance is the big player when it comes to obesity, metabolic syndrome, pre-diabetes, and diabetes type 2. This is the crux of the problem, and where the focus on treatment and a healing protocol needs to be. Insulin resistance precedes diabetes and creates a "metabolic shift." Approximately 25–35% of the population experiences some degree of insulin resistance and suffers the consequences of high blood sugar.[6]

Why is it, then, that we hear about folks losing weight, balancing their blood sugar, and reversing diabetes? On the surface, excess body weight can appear to be the problem behind and the cause of diabetes. But just because events happen at the same time or close together, doesn't make them cause and effect.

You see, when your insulin resistance morphs into insulin sensitivity (when your cells become receptive to insulin and glucose), because you've been tending to your health with a holistic practices, *many* symptoms correct themselves. Weight balances, blood sugar comes into an appropriate zone (fasting blood sugar: 85–100 mg/dL), fatigue does a 360-degree turn, mood swings steady, and energy prevails.

WHITE COATS AND PHYSIOLOGY

Unfortunately, many doctors lag behind the times. Turning a blind eye to current, cutting-edge research, they focus on addressing the symptoms of type 2 diabetes instead of the root cause. Treating symptoms not only gives at best a temporary fix, but it also tends to rely on oral drugs and insulin to force blood sugar down instead of allowing the body to lower it naturally.

(This book, of course, focuses on eradicating diabetes at its root.)

If you experience type 2 diabetes, I guarantee you are not deficient in metformin, nor are you deficient in insulin (as is the case with type 1 diabetes). Instead, your problem is your overexposure to insulin, as it continuously gets pumped out by your pancreas but is unable to move efficiently into your cells.

You experience insulin resistance when your cells have become closed off, despondent, and insensitive to insulin. As a result, the glucose is not granted entry to your cells and stays lingering in your bloodstream. This leads to high blood sugar, which can create a host of negative health conditions. Addressing high blood sugar means addressing the symptom of your condition; addressing insulin resistance means addressing the root.

TREAT HER WELL

Insulin, the hormone secreted by your pancreas post–carbohydrate intake, needs to be treated with respect. At her best, she is a slow and steady traveler. Push her too hard, too often, and she will appear in excess of what your body can handle. This creates an overexposure of insulin, and your cells become weary, losing their appreciation for the traveler on her journey of sugar transport.

Insulin essentially has three jobs:[7]

- Delivering sugar and other calories to your cells for immediate energy.
- Communicating with your liver to convert excess sugar into fat for long-term energy storage.
- Stimulating cell growth.

Processed sugars push her, as do all flour products, grains, and even fruit. Of course, no two body systems are the same, and insulin is going to act differently and uniquely in each case. She hates inactivity, especially hours upon hours of sitting. Feed her right, and she'll treat you well. Neglect her, and you're in for a heap of trouble.

My *Holistic Practices Lifestyle (HPL)* will give you the knowledge, fuel, and inspiration to transform insulin resistance to insulin sensitivity. Along the way, your body weight will balance itself naturally.

HOLISTIC PRACTICES LIFESTYLE

Holistic.
Practices.
Lifestyle.
Holistic. Practices. *Lifestyle*.

This is a mantra I want you to remember. It is your center point, the pathway to preventing and reversing disease and reclaiming joy, vitality, and plenty.

This center point is accomplished by practicing. You will practice. *Practice*.

How is it done? One step, one breath, and one moment at a time.

By developing your own daily holistic practices, and, well, *practicing*, you will learn how to consistently prevent and reverse type 2 diabetes and other conditions. Imagine living with enhanced joy, vitality, and plenty—not to mention the tremendous quality of life you can achieve by awakening your self-confidence and liberating yourself from disease. I'd say that's a pretty good deal, and it's available from nothing more than simple daily practices.

To a large degree, conditions of all sorts—including high blood sugar, high blood pressure, high cholesterol, metabolic syndrome, type 2 diabetes, and heart disease—are a product of your environment and lifestyle. How you deal with stress, what you eat, the extent and way in which you move your body, and how your body handles environmental toxins, are indicative of your level of wellness.[8] This is why I implore you to *practice*.

Healing is not only about bringing physical ailments back into balance. True holistic healing takes place when you pay attention and tend to your entire essence, the whole of who you are—body, mind, and spirit. If you think about it ... when you suffer from symptoms of any disease or imbalance, the anguish is not only in your body; it is also in your mind and spirit.

The good news is that you have incredible influence over the quality of life you are living. When you approach your life holistically through education; belief; a hefty curiosity about the connection between your body, mind, and spirit; and a willingness to take action, it is impossible NOT to change, to transform—to heal. You create an opening, a pathway for bringing your entire system into balance.

ALL 16 PRACTICES, YOU SAY?

Fear not: You do not need to take on every practice in this book. These practices are lifestyle shifts that happen over the long run; choose a few and go deep rather than wide. There's no universal order or best place to start; you must listen to your intuition and grab what you gravitate toward—what you feel inspired by.

That is not to say that some of the practices won't be favorites or that some others won't push you beyond your comfort zone. Make it fun; pick and choose as you like. Mix and match, shake it up, and get creative.

I said there was no best place to start. I'm going to take that back and make a suggestion. I recommend, if you don't already have one, that you start with Practice #8: Create a Morning Ritual.

Here's why: Your morning ritual practice sets the tone and pace of your day. It also begins a domino effect for your other holistic practices. A morning ritual is one of the easier practices to start with and only requires 10 to 15 minutes. Furthermore, it's a practice you design: you decide what to include, the order, style, and so on. It is exactly tailored to you, which can make it easier to follow.

***

Sixteen practices may seem like a lot. While they are all worthy of your time and energy, some won't be a good fit for you, while others will become lifestyle remedies. Behold the spectacular: As you are consistent with a few practices, over time you'll notice yourself doing a greater number of practices than you thought possible, without much added effort.

Call it compound interest: The practices bind and integrate with one another. They take on a rhythm of their own in your new lifestyle—and as a significant part of your new lifestyle. So don't fret about how many practices you start out with or what is ahead of you; dive in with joy. You may be surprised at how many practices you are doing in a short amount of time!

The 16 holistic practices are extensions of these five areas:

1. The Magic of Food: Plants, Herbs, & Nutrients
2. Moving Your Body: The Joy Infusion
3. Stress-Reduction: The Mindset Shift
4. Creative Self-Expression: Your Spirit's Calling
5. Food Addiction: A Social/Emotional Context

These are the five components of my coaching program that I teach to individual clients. These are folks just like you who are ready to expand their vision and mindset, and walk the path to simply feeling better. Inside these five major areas are the branches that connect the dots to a life transformed from *Chaos of Symptoms* to *Symptom Reduction/Elimination* to *Optimal Health*.

Inspire yourself,
Dr. Nicki

MY INTENTION FOR YOU

A FEW UGLY STATISTICS

As of 2016, 29.1 million Americans have been diagnosed with type 2 diabetes. Another 8.1 million have diabetes but are unaware of it. Type 2 diabetes is the 7th leading cause of death in the U.S. As many as 25% of the diabetes population will eventually develop a foot ulcer, and these ulcers precede 85% of lower extremity amputations. Every hour, 10 Americans undergo amputation due to diabetes, and the mortality rate five years post-amputation is approximately 50%.[9]

Did you know that in primitive cultures, conditions such as type 2 diabetes, heart disease, arthritis, cancer, and hypertension are rare?[9] *However, when the same groups of people adopt a Western diet, particularly refined carbohydrates, within one generation, those conditions become rampant.*[10]

Now that we've confronted those hard-to-swallow statistics with open eyes, let's shift course. You, the everyday person, deserve access to the truth about healing, symptom reduction/elimination, and optimal health that has been silenced by the mainstream voice of Western medicine.

WHO IS THE *EVERYDAY PERSON* AND WHY IS THIS IMPORTANT?

You are the everyday person. Whoever you are, whatever your circumstances, this book is for you.

What you do *not* need to heal yourself:

- $10,000 for a diabetes retreat
- a fancy Vitamix high-speed blender
- to take time off of work or away from your family
- to spend hours buried in boring technical medical books or online searches

Your body has an intuitive ability to heal. With the support of life-enhancing practices, healing comes naturally. This book is specifically designed so that regardless of your financial, educational, or social background, you can turn your life around.

Freedom from diabetes is available for everyone. For the everyday person. For *you*.

What you *do* need to heal yourself:

- this book
- a willingness to change your lifestyle
- practice

Congratulations—you're already two-thirds of the way there!

On that note, my intention is to reach folks who may not otherwise have access to this information. If you know someone who needs the information this book has to offer, please spread the word.

PART TWO:
6 MYTHS YOU NEED TO KNOW ABOUT
HEALTH & ILLNESS

WHY START WITH MYTHS?

I feel it's important to address long-held beliefs about health and healing before starting you on your practices. Understanding these myths will help you stand strong against naysayers—and against your doubts. It can be difficult to move forward with new practices if your own beliefs hold you back!

Holding onto misconstrued beliefs—that is, thoughts set in concrete that are simply not true—is a great way to stay stuck in unmanageable patterns of addiction: terrifying food behaviors that seem to have a hold on you, lethargy, and disease.

Sometimes, you simply need to be given permission to stop believing old, outdated, and harmful beliefs. Give yourself permission! Educate and re-educate yourself. Let me be your guide and lend a hand by pointing out new and improved research, life- and health-affirming beliefs, and substantiated commonsense factors to live by.

MYTH #1: IT'S OKAY TO INGEST CHEMICALS

The actual amount of filth and waste, which is the "mysterious" cause of your "trouble," is almost unbelievable.

—Arnold Ehret, PhD

In an insidious fashion, chemical additives (which I'll hereafter simply call "chemicals") are embedded in our food, nutritional supplements, cleaning products, cosmetics, linens, clothes, mattresses … and the list goes on. You must become a master inspector and choose wisely to avoid the injury of these endocrine disrupters. According to the National Institute of Environmental Health Sciences:

> Endocrine disruptors are chemicals that may interfere with the body's endocrine system and produce adverse developmental, reproductive, neurological, and immune effects in both humans and wildlife. A wide range of substances, both natural and man-made, are thought to cause endocrine disruption, including pharma-

ceuticals, dioxin and dioxin-like compounds, polychlorinated biphenyls, DDT and other pesticides, and plasticizers such as bisphenol A. Endocrine disruptors may be found in many everyday products—including plastic bottles, metal food cans, detergents, flame retardants, food, toys, cosmetics, and pesticides.[11]

In other words: Many chemicals found in common products alter your immune and nervous systems and degrade cell function.

Your body is not meant to ingest or process chemicals; the correlation between a rise in chronic illness and the increase of manmade chemicals in our food and other supplies proves it.[12] Collectively, the more we move away from whole foods in their unprocessed state and toward food-like products, the sicker we become.

So why hasn't this correlation been more publicized? Why isn't it on labels? Why do so many manufacturers tell us to focus on macronutrients—fats, protein, and carbohydrates? Because they know that if red dye #3, blue dye #4, and other (mostly unpronounceable) chemicals were highlighted on food packages, their sales would plummet.

Food is not the only concern; nutritional supplements are not immune from fooling everyday people. In fact, nutritional supplements are a multi-billion-dollar industry[13] where greed reigns king. Just like food, not all supplements are created equal. You generally need to search far and wide to find a clean supplement—that is, one without fillers such as magnesium stearate, vegetable stearate, silica, and soy lecithin.

The learning curve to becoming a master inspector for whole vs. chemical-laden ingredients is well worth your effort. Chemical additives should be the first thing you cut from your food plan, 100%, with no exceptions.

ON A PERSONAL NOTE

I have a purposeful habit of smelling household items in the store before I buy them. The type and degree of the scent gives me an indication of the level of chemical toxicity in the product or packaging. If I inhale a whiff of that distinctive, unpleasant smell ... back on the shelf it goes.

Some synthetic aromas are initially hidden, only to be discovered later. Sometimes it's not the scent at all, but rather, the effect on my health that I notice. This comes in the way of headaches (which I rarely get), fatigue, or feeling lousy all over—much like having the flu.

I have driven myself near crazy with constant smelling, trying to determine if a scent is synthetic or natural. The extent of chemical-culture has definitely had an impact on my life. Just consider the time it has cost me on the research alone, even before all the sniffing and analyzing!

The best solution I've found is shopping in natural, eco-friendly stores. I do this as much as possible, whenever I can. However, since it's not always possible, don't be surprised if you bump into me while sniffing my way through the aisles at World Market; Target; or Bed, Bath, & Beyond.

MYTH #2: EATING DIETARY FAT & CHOLESTEROL WILL MAKE YOU FAT

In the last half century, the US government prescription of a low- to no-fat diet to prevent heart disease, obesity and diabetes has failed. Current studies showing epidemic and continued rising numbers in obesity and type 2 diabetes have shown the low-fat recommendation to be dangerous to body, mind, and spirit.

—California Superfood Chef

This myth is responsible for the fat-free revolution, which has helped to create an epidemic of obesity. What makes it worse is that when fat is removed from food, sugar is typically increased. For decades, this has sent us into a tailspin of carbohydrate overload. The truth is that only 5% to 10% of dietary cholesterol makes up your blood cholesterol. Cholesterol is made by your liver, and is ultra-important for producing cell membranes, hormones, and vitamin D.

If the macronutrient we typically call fat were called by its technical name, lipid,[*] we might not be so confused. It's faulty to think that eating fat makes you fat. The misinformation fad all started with misguided research in the late 1950s by Ancel Keys.[14] This unsound research led us to believe that dietary fat and cholesterol were villains. **This was one of the biggest mistakes in the history of health and nutrition.** It has done great harm, and we will be unraveling it for years to come.

The medical industry is slowly catching up and being forced to pay attention to current research—how fat and cholesterol *actually* affect health. Sadly, some folks will never change their beliefs. This myth has simply been ingrained too long for some to explore a new reality.

You might wonder who's benefited from consuming little to no fat and cholesterol. It certainly hasn't been the American people. The problem is that if you don't go down one road, you travel down another. If you're not satiated from healthy fats and proteins, you're eventually going to crash into *Carbohydrate Lane.*

Carbohydrate Lane isn't typically filled with veggies and low-glycemic fruit; instead, it houses fast-converting-to-sugar carbs, such as grain flours (bread, cookies, crackers, pretzels, etc.) and simple sugar desserts. This is where you need a big, red alert sign that says, *Choose Your Carbohydrates Wisely.*

You see, it isn't the cholesterol and fat you eat that mostly determine your cholesterol levels, ratio of good to bad cholesterol, and excess fat in your bloodstream; it's the sugar and starches you eat.[15]

Take this to heart: increased nut and seed (raw, unsalted) consumption is associated with a lower risk of type 2 diabetes and heart disease. [16] Not eating nuts and seeds because they are

---

[*] Fats (technically called triglycerides) are actually a subcategory of the macronutrient lipid. I use "fat" because this is the word most people are familiar with.

"fattening" is one of the worst pieces of advice ever offered to the American public.[17]

ON A PERSONAL NOTE

I grew up in the 1970s' low-fat, no-fat craze, both inside my house and out. My mother still lives in that craze. No fault of hers; like many people, she has not deconstructed the fat-myth derived many years ago from faulty research. Imagine, if you would, dissecting a food and yanking out one of its main components: fat. Truly a non-holistic move.

You can't do that with whole foods, can you? This is why I gravitate toward eating carrots, red bell peppers, avocados, pastured eggs, berries, and grapefruits, etc. Let's see how long it takes the scientists to make low-fat avocados. Ridiculous!

For me, the big *stay-away-from* food is sugar, not fat. While the word "sugar" may provoke visions of colorful desserts, it also includes flour products. I have said many times (from my unconscious place): "Send me to an island with sprouted, seeded whole-grain fresh bread and organic grass-fed butter or extra virgin olive oil, and I'll be happy!" Of course, I would not survive too long on the flour's empty-nutrient, high-glycemic calories. The fat would help slow down the sugar conversion of the bread, but my blood sugar would still be high, and my intestines wouldn't be thrilled.

MYTH #3: TRUST YOUR DOCTOR NO MATTER WHAT

I want to talk to you about one of the biggest myths in medicine, and that is the idea that all we need are more medical breakthroughs and then all of our problems will be solved.

—Dr. Quyen Nguyen

Have you handed the destiny of your health to your doctor?

Is your doctor a healer?

I caution you: do not relinquish your power to a doctor without having gained trust in her or his ability to reach for the source of your imbalance. **If your doctor is merely treating symptoms, step away and find someone else.** Focusing on symptom reduction through a chemical approach is a Band-Aid technique.

In fact, you need not give away your power at all. First, you'll need to see yourself as a co-participant in your healthcare, in order to advocate for yourself. Then and only then, partner with a practitioner who treats you as a co-participant. Find a healer whose method is to reach below the surface of the symptom, keeping your long-term recovery top-of-mind.

Doctors in traditional medical schools receive very little education on nutrition—imagine that. We know that food is information,[18] not merely calories. If your doctor/healer/practitioner is not monitoring how this information affects YOU, he or she is likely doing you a disservice.

If your doctor/healer/practitioner is quickly flipping you chemical pharmaceuticals in the hopes of masking symptoms, rather than getting to the source of distress, she/he is consciously or unconsciously doing you harm.

It's important you know your doctor's approach or philosophy about health, illness, and medicine. What a concept, right? And speaking of rights, it is your *right as a patient* to know your doctor's approach. Do not move blindly into any kind of healthcare treatment without knowing what you are agreeing to.

Your best tool is asking your practitioner questions—lots of questions. If she seems reluctant or defensive, find a new doctor. Find someone down-to-earth who speaks your language, who is aligned with your mindset. Do not settle for second best ... ever.

ON A PERSONAL NOTE

There were so many times I went with the flow of the man or woman in the white coat.

Two pap smears come to mind, so let's go there. The first occasion was in Southern California. I was literally kicking the wall in front of me due to the pain. The doctor didn't slow down or show any emotional expression to this. The second occasion was in San Francisco. There, the nurse practitioner did not know what she was doing, and left me bleeding.

Flashback to a childhood memory at Kaiser Hospital in Los Angeles. My left ear was clogged with wax (I swam in pools a lot), which the doctor proceeded to stick a long metal object down my ear to remove. My mother, who was sitting beside me, felt the pain too, and shuddered at the unnerving procedure. Many years later, I found a gentle nurse practitioner at Sutter East Bay Medical Foundation in Berkeley, CA, who skillfully and painlessly performed the same procedure (with a non-metal device). When I tell you it was almost pleasurable, I kid you not.

Then there was a Los Angeles body check for moles. While removing a couple of skin tags (benign out-pouchings of skin), the dermatologist said with a nasty tone, "You just know how to grow these things." Hmmm, that wasn't a warm, fuzzy moment.

Most recently, in Santa Cruz, CA, I had a cardiologist check-up post coronary artery stent (tiny wire mesh tube) placement. The physician's assistant gave me a 20-minute, monotone narrative recommending chemical medicines void of ANY lifestyle practices, thoughts, ideas, or suggestions. Glazed over, I made short vocal sounds, acknowledging her with one-word responses. It was all I could do to get through the appointment. I wish, I wish ... upon a star ... that I had said, "This isn't a good fit for me," and rescheduled with a different practitioner. Her medicine wasn't *my* medicine; it wasn't integrative in the least.

MYTH #4: THERE IS A ONE-SIZE-FITS-ALL IN NUTRITION

The art of healing comes from nature and not from the physician. Therefore, the physician must start from nature with an open mind.

—Paracelsus

Too much fruit, not enough fruit, high healthy-fats, high carb, low carb, vegan, raw, paleo, intermittent fasting, three meals a day or six ... **the best food plan is the one that's right for YOU.** You can learn from teachers and study the research, but ultimately, you'll need to weed through it, experiment, and listen fiercely to your body and intuition. You are your own best expert!

If anyone tells you there is a one-size-fits-all when it comes to nutrition and health, run the other way.

As a human being, you are part of a species made up of a variety of subtle as well as obvious differences. The differences in how your body responds on a cellular level to food, movement, and stress set you apart from everyone else. It's certainly true: you are unique. It's therefore simply foolish for a practitioner, health coach, doctor, or other guide to give you a predetermined treatment formula. Devising a one-size-fits-all nutrition plan is easy, but, quite frankly, it is unethical. Getting your nutrition right is a process. It's an evolution of trial and error, experimentation, and experience.

For example: Why is it that you can easily digest a type of food your friend cannot? Why is your friend's blood sugar level not even close to pre-diabetic as you watch her enjoy sugar-laden desserts? Meanwhile, a simple piece of tropical fruit knocks your blood sugar out of whack. The answer is simple: You do not process ingredients the same way your "brothers and sisters" do.

Do not compare yourself to anyone else. Yes, it's easier said than done, and that's why I'm telling you now: to give you a head start. Seek to discover the nutrition plan that serves you best.

ON A PERSONAL NOTE

Certain perspectives in raw vegan culture would have me eating buckets of fruit, any fruit, all day, every day. I've had folks tell me personally this was the absolute best way to eat—diabetic or not, insulin-resistant or not. This blatantly false belief is the kind of one-size-fits-all approach to nutrition that I find absolutely absurd. You see, we all process sugar differently, so while some people can handle buckets of fruit, this would be a path of destruction for me.

At a lecture in Berkeley, CA, I absorbed the teachings of Dr. Brian Clement, director of the *Hippocrates Health Institute,* in West Palm Beach, FL. He spoke about the profound health benefits of raw foods and veggie juicing. He also said that when he travels for speaking engagements, which he does quite a bit, he makes allowances in his meal plan. He said he did his best, but food was not his religion. Similarly, I attempt to do my best to integrate flexibility in my meal plan.

Reflecting on a moment I'd eaten a flour/sugar concoction, it was easy to get down on myself. Maybe you know that negative, demeaning self-talk I'm thinking about? Luckily, I became aware of a concept from wise author and teacher Eckhart Tolle: "Is there any problem in *this* moment?" As usual, the answer was "no"—and I continued onward.

MYTH #5: FOOD PACKAGES AREN'T MISLEADING

The single biggest health problem we face globally is the metabolic disaster that has led to a global epidemic of obesity, type 2 diabetes, and heart disease.

—Dr. Mark Hyman

"Wholesome, natural, healthy, organic…" The writing on the front of food packages is marketing, meant to sell you products. Pull out your inspector glasses and turn the package over. While it's tempting to focus on the macronutrient label (protein, fats, and carbohydrates), this can prevent you from seeing the bigger picture.

Is your health at the forefront of the manufacturer's mind? Perhaps not. Think sales … lots of sales. Notice the shiny words and descriptions that get you to pick up and buy the product—"organic, pure, fresh, no sugar, non-GMO, low sugar, low-fat." How about "gluten-free"?

Packaging is marketing, my friends. Marketing is big business, *really* BIG business, producing masses of money. The object of marketing is to sell you the product. That means the smart manufacturer is going to make the packaging as enticing and attractive to you, the consumer, as possible.

Organic doesn't necessarily mean 100% organic, and non-GMO (non-genetically modified organism) doesn't mean organic. Wholesome—what is that? Weren't we told Wonder Bread was wholesome? "Heart-healthy" by whose guidelines? If you blindly trust marketing gimmicks on labels, you may be easily fooled.

Instead, move your eyes to the list of ingredients. Notice what is actually in the product you're about to eat. How much of it is food you can identify? What about chemicals and additives? Use your wisdom to determine if it's best left on the shelf.

Adjust your inspector glasses to find fantastic, good-for-you products. They are made by health-focused brands with integrity that have *your* health at the forefront of their hearts and minds.

Now turn that package over and read the list of ingredients!

ON A PERSONAL NOTE

I don't know about you, but sometimes I turn a blind eye and re-main in denial. I want to believe and trust packaging because I want to eat the [fill in the blank—usually a flour/sugar get-together]. "Please don't tell me this food has inflammatory oils such as canola and safflower. Please don't tell me agave syrup (a highly processed nightmare) is the sweetener." Sometimes, I just don't want to know.

It's easy to fool myself, especially at a party or gathering where the goods are out of their suspicious packages, already resting in bowls. I simply tell myself what I want to hear; how convenient.

Sometimes, I know the truth and indulge anyway. I end up pay-ing for it by way of a bloated belly, inflamed gut, exhaustion, high blood sugar, extreme crash, or foggy mood.

The point, however, is while we might not always eat properly, we can at least prevent ourselves from eating improperly through ignorance—by educating ourselves enough to *not* be fooled by clever marketing.

Choose wisely.

MYTH #6: GLUTEN-FREE MEANS HEALTHY

> The popularity of the gluten-free diet has given rise to an industry of gluten-free convenience foods that contain questionable additives, added sugar, and nutrient-empty ingredients.
>
> —Vani Hari

Dr. William Davis, author of *Wheat Belly*, said, "Be gluten-free but don't eat gluten-free," for good reason.[19] If you haven't noticed, the gluten-free craze has blown up across the nation. This bigtime industry does not always have your best interests at heart.

Many alternative flours used in gluten-free products (cornstarch, potato starch, rice starch, tapioca flour, etc.) are high-glycemic, addicting, and just as inflammatory as wheat.

Gluten-free is not a green flag to devour muffins and flour products to your heart's content. Wrap yourself around this concept: You must know what you are eating; gluten-free only tells you what you *aren't* eating—gluten.

How you use the gluten-free phenomenon is up to you, and this decision will make a difference between getting healthier and getting sicker. If you're running to the muffin aisle (and I know this well) for those wheat-free goodies, you may want to slow down and recognize what you're running toward.

Ask yourself these questions: Are those fluffy flour-bombs going to increase, improve, and support my health, or are they going to hinder my progress? How will I feel after eating them? Do I secretly know I am addicted and using gluten-free products in the exact same way I consumed their wheat-laden cousins? Have I simply switched my addiction from one crappy food-like product to another?

What are the healthier alternatives to wheat, barley, rye, cornstarch, rice starch, potato starch, and tapioca flour? Almond and coconut flour, and some folks tolerate quinoa or millet flour.

ON A PERSONAL NOTE

Though I know it isn't great for me, I find bread delightfully satiating and enjoyable.

Initially when the gluten-free craze began, I made the transition from wheat to all types of gluten-free products: bread, bagels, muffins, cookies, cakes, pretzels—you name it. If only heaven existed in those scrumptious, gooey, gluten-free lovelies! But it didn't.

Fast forward a few years to when I was ready to get honest with myself. I did the research. Based on my belief of being my own best guide—needing to listen to my body signals and intuitive cues—I started exploring my own well of wisdom. It wasn't hard to determine that I didn't feel well. Digestion reveals all.

I discovered that most gluten-free products are made with incredibly crappy ingredients. Starches, oils, and sugars that spiked my blood sugar, tied my belly in knots (hello, inflammation, the root cause of illness), left me feeling foggy and addicted, and weighed heavily on my heart—figuratively and literally.

My meal plan is an ongoing negotiation between my mind and

my awareness. I make my best choices when I am satiated. If I am starving or quickly dropping into a blood-sugar low while passing a bakery, street café, or the baked goods section of my local natural grocer … wish me luck.

PART THREE: 16 HOLISTIC PRACTICES

BEFORE YOU DIVE IN...

The *Holistic Practices Lifestyle* can be applied to many illnesses and no illness; to physical, mental, and emotional imbalances; and no imbalance. It can be used as prevention to guard against ill health, or implemented to simply make your life better—more enjoyable; even invigorating. When you follow along and practice, you may lose sight of diabetes and sickness altogether.

If you feel tempted to cling, to reach back to illness and hold it tightly in your grip, know this is a learned state, a place of familiarity. Here's the thing: If you're practicing, you are on the right track. You don't need to stay focused on imbalance, disease, or type 2 diabetes to heal yourself.

Where is the quick fix to fantastic health? You won't find it here, because it doesn't exist. There is no quick-fix cure—natural or chemical. Practicing is a long-term game. You are here for the long run, or you are not here at all.

However, don't take the connection between holistic practices and diabetes lightly—lifestyle intervention is often more effective in reducing diabetes, heart disease, stroke, cancer, hypertension, and death than almost any other medical intervention.[20]

For easy access and quick reference, I recommend you refer to my **supplemental companion guides** as you move through the practices. You'll find them on my resources page.[*]

---

[*] http://drnickisteinberger.com/waveresources

ON A PERSONAL NOTE

When I reversed diabetes, I had a handful of the 16 practices in my bag, but certainly not all. It has taken me a number of years to develop the entire lot, test them by trial and error, discard some, and keep the rest.

I have called upon patience, diligence, and surrender to find what works best for me. Once I solidified the practices, I started sharing them with family and friends, and then teaching clients, community workshops, universities, and business trainings.

The practices are alive in the sense that they are ever-evolving. They are not my religion; they are signposts on my path. I travel with them as long as they serve me well and say goodbye as my body and intuition suggest.

Some of these practices were instrumental in reversing type 2 diabetes, while others were brewing just ahead of me on the path, waiting for my arrival. There is life after diabetes—good life, simple life.

Whether I am practicing in a prevention state or a reversal state, the work and focus are the same. If I fall, I pick myself up, dust off my pants, and get to walking or meditating or hydrating or increasing my intake of healthy fats or whatever else needs doing.

PRACTICE #1: DRINK WATER WITH LEMON UPON RISING

Even the most winged spirit cannot escape
physical necessity.

—Kahlil Gibran

The first substance you consume in the morning needs to be water. This will hydrate your system immediately and wake you up on a cellular level. Throughout the day, continue to drink approximately 1/2 your body weight in ounces of water (e.g., if you weigh 180 lbs, drink 90 ounces of pure water daily).

Adding fresh squeezed lemon to your water will create an alkalizing process that reduces inflammation. Inflammation is a root cause of almost all chronic diseases, including type 2 diabetes, heart disease, and cancer.[21] Though lemon is an acidic fruit, it is alkalizing when eaten.

As you sleep, swelling occurs.[22] This is why you may wake up congested, groggy, with sleep in your eyes, and slow-moving. This clogging also occurs inside your body. After all, your organs, bloodstream, and cells have been lying still for hours. It's a susceptible time for inflammation.

The healthiest first-thing-in-the-morning practice is flushing your system. Help your body move the toxins that have accumulated overnight. It's a simple practice, to start your day with a glass of fresh water and hand-squeezed lemon. It's a smart idea to make this your beverage of choice, before reaching for coffee, tea, or food.

Remember, you are breaking a fast each morning. Since you aren't eating while sleeping, your body, organs, blood, and cells finally get to rest. Doesn't it make sense to allow your insides to wake up slowly? Slow awakening and cleansing are what happen when you flush your system and then gradually introduce other ingredients—beverages and food.

Hydrating with fresh lemon upon rising feels so good, too—clean, pure, and in right alignment. This practice allows you to start your day with multiple health benefits—hydration, inflammation-reduction, toxin-cleansing and purification, vitamin C nourishment, and the list goes on.

ON A PERSONAL NOTE

In my morning hydration practice, I interchange fresh-squeezed lemon with a capful of apple cider vinegar (ACV: great for balancing blood sugar) in my glass of room-temperature water. I drink diligently. Why? Because along with the known health benefits, my body responds positively to the cool splash.

I cannot imagine eating before I plunge into my water source. Even meditation comes after hydration. This is my first self-care practice of the day, every day. I emphasize the daily aspect of it because consistency is the key element in practicing. Success builds over time; success is cumulative.

My body and intuition tell me that hydrating as my first practice of the day is a non-optional necessity. Whether I choose fresh lemon or ACV, I feel the cleansing effects almost immediately. Day after day, this practice supports my digestion and assists me in meeting the day with full presence.

What is your first practice of the day? How does it support you?

PRACTICE #2: MEDITATE A MINIMUM OF 10 MINUTES EVERY DAY

Feelings come and go like clouds in a windy sky.
Conscious breathing is my anchor.
—Thich Nhat Hanh

You may have heard that meditation is powerful medicine. Without question, the transformative effects meditation has on the body, mind, and spirit are profound.[23]

Meditation dates back to 1500 BCE and has been a significant part of nearly every religious practice. That tells us the benefits of meditation are grounded in experience. You need not be religious to receive the health benefits of meditation.

Meditating is a remarkably holistic practice, because it impacts your entire essence—the whole of who you are—body, mind, and spirit.

As you meditate, your body relaxes. You engage your parasympathetic nervous system,[24] reducing your stress-response, and enhancing a state of calm. Body functions such as digestion and heart rate are supported in a slow and gentle way.

During meditation, the thinking mind gets quiet; this is beneficial, considering life is filled with chatter. Incessant thinking can be overwhelming and stressful. Giving yourself a break from thinking is relaxing and whisks you away from the chaotic mind-play you may find yourself bathed in, possibly chained to throughout the day.

Meditating lifts your spirit. It does this by allowing you to be present, which is a gift. You see, as you meditate, you come into alignment with the part of you that is pure and simple awareness—consciousness, if you will. *Presence* is peaceful and still, merely witnessing or catching a glimpse of the ego-body/thinking-mind rambling forward.

This practice will bring you closer to who you are. It clears the dust.

Take a "dose" first thing in the morning and throughout the day as needed. You can meditate alone in a sacred nook or with a group of peace-seekers in a meditation center or other group setting.

ON A PERSONAL NOTE

For a long time, I didn't understand meditation. I knew it was beneficial, and that it had passed through the ages as an ancient holy ritual. I knew folks swore by it as their center point for daily grounding. It wasn't until I embodied the significance of being present—of bringing my consciousness to the present time as a moment-by-moment practice—that the value of meditation as a tool became crystal clear.

Now, I approach my meditation practice from the standpoint of practicing presence. I know that when I meditate, I will be giving myself a chance to awaken to the moment of now, whether my meditation lasts for 5 minutes or 20. It is a place where I get to remember who I am. If this seems odd, esoteric, or confusing, I suggest reading *A New Earth* by Eckhart Tolle, as it changed my life.

Starting my day without meditating feels like something went missing. It happens at times, and I don't beat myself up over it. I do, however, feel a slight longing, as if waving goodbye to a moment passed.

My meditation practice (which, by the way, comes right after Practice #1: Drink Water with Lemon upon Rising) begins with sound—listening to and quietly naming the sounds I hear: bird, car, fan, walking, etc. This brings me back to center and reminds me why I am here (presence). From there, I entertain affirmation, visualization, inspirational reading, and scribing (writing in my journal).

I purchased special pillows to sit on in an area I call my meditation corner. It's cozy, comfy, and pretty; it's inviting. In front of me are large windows with huge pines and a massive hilly ridge in the distance. This is quite settling, tranquil, and primitive.

As lovely as my designated mediation corner is, I don't let being away from its familiarity stop me from my practice. I do my best to meditate wherever I am. No bells or whistles needed.

PRACTICE #3: DECREASE OR ELIMINATE FAST-CONVERTING CARBOHYDRATES

I told the doctor I broke my leg in two places.
He told me to quit going to those places.
—Henry Youngman

As is the case with fats and protein, there is diversity among carbohydrates. The source of a carbohydrate determines its benefit or detriment. You can be absolutely sure you need carbs to survive and thrive, as they are an important source of energy to your cells, but you need to choose wisely.

Let me interrupt all assumption that carbohydrates are bad or to be avoided at all costs. Macronutrient lesson 101: Carbohydrates, fats, and proteins are all necessary. Removing or severely limiting any of these macronutrients is a short-term approach that will not produce successful, long-term results.

Let's take a deeper look.

Carbs turn to sugar in your bloodstream. This is a normal process, so don't be afraid of it; instead, act smartly. Your pancreas releases insulin, the hormone that grabs the sugar from your blood-stream and transports it to your cells. This is one way energy is created, giving you the get-up-and-go you need to do your thing.

However, it's not beneficial to send insulin out urgently multiple times a day due to an excess of blood-sugar spikes. Think of insulin as your friend, and don't run her down, or else you'll burn her out. Your pancreas can become weak and tired if it works too hard sending insulin out to save the day over and over again.

Fast-converting carbohydrates turn to sugar quickly when they hit your bloodstream; this causes a spike in blood sugar, and will send you on an up-down spiral. This reaction is one piece of the puzzle that paves the way to metabolic syndrome, pre-diabetes, and type 2 diabetes.[25]

Stay clear of these fast-converting-carbohydrate speed demons: processed sugars, grain flours (wheat, rye, barley, rice starch, potato starch, corn starch, tapioca flour), breads, bagels, cookies, pretzels, pancakes, pizza, cake, candy, rice, white potatoes, and some fruit such as dates and other high-glycemic fruit.

On the other hand, enjoy the delicious, sustained energy and health benefits of slow-converting-to-sugar carbs, your friends: vegetables, leafy greens, berries, limited beans and legumes.

ON A PERSONAL NOTE

I want to emphasize that for many of us, me included, decreasing or eliminating fast-converting, high-sugar carbs is not merely about mindset or making a decision. Success requires practice; that is to say, there are ups and downs, highs an lows. Though *you* may be able to simply make this decision and stick to it, *I* find myself riding the slow-carb train a lot of the time, and the fast-carb train some of the time. I have not mastered this practice by any means.

Fast-converting carbs, particularly bread products and desserts, lure me in. Maybe you can relate to the feeling of instant gratification? I'm not going to hide or sugarcoat how this addiction has impacted my life.

If I peek behind my own veil, I see type 2 diabetes, metabolic syndrome, and heart disease. Paving the way was high LDL cholesterol, high blood sugar, mood swings, irritability, fatigue, distancing myself from others, anger, and isolation. All this from seemingly harmless vegan chocolate donuts, veggie burgers, sweetened chai lattes, the stress of graduate school, and organic, sprouted, whole-grain bread.

When I'm clean, I'm clean. While there are many theories on cravings, I can generally expect a measurable dissipation of my cravings within 30 days of eliminating specific ingredients. I have experienced this with sugar and flour many times. Unfortunately, once the same ingredients are reintroduced to my meal plan, I am back in the saddle again.

Here is a helpful list of addiction zappers in no particular order:

- Support from a close friend
- Overeaters Anonymous (OA) meetings
- Knowing my healthier alternative choices
- Stocking up on my healthier alternative choices
- Moving my body regularly (in nature)
- Veggie juicing daily
- Lots of delicious raw foods
- Increasing my intake of healthy fats and protein
- Meditating
- Gratitude practice
- Self-forgiveness
- Teaching these practices to others

Be gentle with yourself; we're in this together for the long run.

PRACTICE #4: ELIMINATE RANCID & OXIDIZED VEGETABLE OILS

> The food you eat can either be the safest and most powerful form of medicine or the slowest form of poison.
>
> —Dr. Anne Wigmore

Rancid and oxidized oils have been infiltrating our food ecosystem for decades, and they are extremely dangerous. This happened in great part due to the no-fat/low-fat faulty research that sent us headfirst into a bucket of margarine and led us to believe that canola oil was a health food.[26]

These food-like products are not food at all. Margarine is one step away from plastic, and canola oil (from the rapeseed plant) is heavily processed and bleached to remove the awful stench it gives off. Reducing consumption of these oils is not enough. I suggest you run very quickly in the opposite direction, or your liver is likely to pay the price. Also included: storing unwanted, unneeded, and unnecessary visceral fat.[27]

One of the biggest dangers to our collective wellness is rancid and oxidized vegetable oils. These cheaply made, highly processed oils have been extracted from plants, sometimes using a harmful chemical, hexane, in the extraction process. Listen up: your body does not know how to digest these oils, as they were never meant to be food.

Soy oil, corn oil, safflower oil, sunflower oil, canola oil, "vegetable oil," and even olive oil blends are inflammatory. Remember: inflammation and toxicity are root causes of disease. These omega-6 based oils are inflammatory, and need to be avoided.[28]

Vegetable oils and oil blends are literally everywhere. Go ahead, ask your server at the restaurant what kind of oils they use. If she happens to say olive oil, ask if it's a blend. Many restaurants use a blend of olive and canola oil because it's cheaper than using 100% extra virgin olive oil. They take a liberty by calling their blend "olive oil."

Next time you eat at a hot bar (even from your so-called health-food-focused local grocery store), look at the ingredients in the dishes. If they are not listed, ask. You may be amazed at how canola and other health-deflating oils have found their way into numerous foods.

ON A PERSONAL NOTE

At my neighborhood co-op, fresh doughnuts from a local baker arrive Monday, Wednesday, and Friday. Numerous colorful varieties look perky and ready for consumption as they sit upright in their square-shaped, see-through bin. Just because these goodies are vegan doesn't mean they're healthy. Remember Myth #5: "Food Packages Aren't Misleading"? It's marketing, marketing, marketing.

Reading the list of ingredients informs me they are high-quality *compared* to a mainstream local doughnut shop. First of all, the baker only used a handful of ingredients, with no added chemicals or fillers. However, gosh darn it, these sweet treats are made with non-GMO canola oil!

Time permitting, I could add a task to my to-do list to call the baker, express my concerns, and request a healthier oil—coconut perhaps (this works well for baking desserts better than olive oil; I have an olive-oil-cake-replacement-disaster story I'll tell ya some-day).

You may be thinking the "non-GMO" part is good, and it is certainly better than genetically modified canola oil. But that doesn't make it a healthy food or okay for consumption.

Though I am left with an aftertaste I can identify as oil, I don't feel sick after eating one (or two) donuts, but I know it's causing unnoticeable damage. I'm smart enough to know (after all, I've done my research!) that invisible damage on the outside doesn't equate to no harm on the inside—e.g., to my organs and blood. Call it what it is: tasty, destructive inflammation.

PRACTICE #5: INCREASE HEALTHY FATS (YES, DO IT)

> Saturated fats are the preferred fuel for your heart, and are also used as a source of fuel during energy expenditure.
>
> —Dr. Joseph Mercola

Increasing dietary fat intake goes against the mainstream attitude of "stay away." We cannot rewind the fat myth created decades ago by faulty research, but we can wise up now:

Your brain, heart, and multiple body functions need plenty of healthy fats to help you operate optimally and efficiently.[29]

Healthy fats are anti-inflammatory (the least inflammatory macronutrient when compared to protein and carbohydrates) and satiating. Your nerves are lined with fat (myelin), which allows electricity to flow effectively. Do not take this lightly. Saturated fats are the most stable (least likely to oxidize) fat; foods with saturated fat include grass-fed butter, ghee, coconut oil, nuts, seeds, and fatty fish such as salmon and sardines.

Monounsaturated fats (fats that have only one bond) are also healthy; these foods include avocados, olives, extra virgin olive oil, and nuts and seeds—such as almonds, pistachios, and pumpkin seeds.

Your brain is made up of approximately 60 percent fat. Not eating sufficient healthy fats can deteriorate healthy brain function, leading to cognitive decline.[30]

Each meal you eat should include healthy fats. You will feel fuller faster and stay satiated longer. They have a grounding effect as well, so if you need brain energy to work, produce, or create, the fat-stop is the place to fuel up.

Need snacks between meals? Not a problem. Keep your kitchen, car, bike, purse, or backpack stocked with nuts and seeds. Go for almonds, walnuts, brazil nuts, hazelnuts, sunflower seeds, pumpkin seeds, and macadamia nuts. Make sure they're raw, and organic if possible, with nothing added.

Once you start eating greater amounts of healthy fats, you'll feel that sustained, grounded energy and understand why relying on this food group as a daily staple is an excellent choice. There is no one-size-fits-all approach, but more and more folks are experiencing improved blood sugar levels by making this significant adjustment to their meal plan.[31]

ON A PERSONAL NOTE

When I set out to reverse type 2 diabetes the first time in 2010, I was extremely fortunate to have California Superfood Chef by my side. At times, I thought she sounded like a broken record, playing the healthy-fat monologue. Her song ended up being a blessing; her persistence was a response to my resistance.

If you feel resistant yourself, I understand, because I've been there. California Superfood Chef opened my eyes to what I could not see myself. I was primarily focused on veggie juicing and raw foods at the time; that was my jam (I first heard "jam" being used this way by Danielle LaPorte; I quite like it). However powerful the mighty green leaves were, they were only one side of the equation.

My guides—that is, body and intuition—primarily pointed me in one direction: juicing and raw foods. It was a direction I could follow, because it made sense to me, but it was important for me to stay open to the teachers around me. I could not see every angle necessary to heal myself; we rarely do.

I added an abundance of healthy fats to my meals: avocados, raw nuts and seeds (including hemp and chia), grass-fed butter and eggs, and wild salmon. Now, seven years later, healthy-fat research has sprung from the depths, sprinkling its light on the masses.

While this continues to be a controversial topic, my advice as always is to listen to your body and intuition, pay close attention to current research, and experiment. We are our own best teachers.

PRACTICE #6: WRAP CARBOHYDRATES IN FIBER (COMBINATIONS MATTER)

> Foods with more fiber have a lesser effect on blood sugar, and thus have fewer net carbs, whereas foods with little or no fiber but many carbs will cause more of a dramatic increase of your blood glucose.
>
> —Dr. Sara Gottfried

To prevent and reverse type 2 diabetes, it's critical that you slow down the rate of sugar conversion in your bloodstream. When you eat or drink carbohydrates, sugar is released into your blood and then carried by way of insulin to your cells. This produces fuel for energy.

The more slowly carbohydrates convert into sugar, the steadier your blood-sugar balance will be. This supports insulin sensitivity (which is what you want: the opposite of insulin resistance). Rather than remove carbohydrates altogether (which may be easier said than done), you can slow down the rate at which they convert to sugar in your bloodstream by pairing them with fiber.

Surrounding your starchy carbs with fiber will naturally slow down the sugar conversion; on the other hand, combining carbs with proteins or fats will elevate blood sugar and insulin levels.

A piece of fruit will convert to sugar more slowly than a candy bar because it's wrapped in its own natural fruit fiber skin. Potatoes alone will convert faster than potatoes eaten with vegetables (fiber), but once you add the grass-fed butter, coconut oil (fat), or protein (plant or animal), your insulin levels will spike.

Let this practice of food combining bring a smile to your carbohydrate worries. Rather than eliminating carbs completely, pay attention to the types of foods you're combining them with. Instead of thinking you can't have a potato because of the glycemic index and load, eat half of a *sweet potato*, boil instead of bake, and include a mound of leafy greens and plenty of non-starchy vegetables.

Think of this as a puzzle, and identify where the pieces fit. In this equation, notice what's missing and where you can fill in the blanks. I suggest keeping it simple for ease, fun, and success. Carbs plus veggies—green light, go. Carbs plus fat and protein—red light, stop.

When it comes to fats and proteins, go ahead and eat them together. Toss a handful of raw nuts or seeds on your plate; add avocado and greens, extra virgin olive oil, and choose your protein source—plant or animal. Smart combining allows you to enjoy a full spectrum of ingredients with an insulin-friendly approach.

ON A PERSONAL NOTE

Creating balance in my meals—breakfast, lunch, dinner, and snacks—became easier when I started implementing the practice of surrounding any fast-converting-to-sugar carbohydrates I ate with foods that were high in fiber.

This also simplified meal decision-making and prep-time coordination. I knew if I was having any kind of starchy carbohydrate, I needed to *surround* it with non-starchy vegetables, leafy greens, and fresh herbs but *leave out* the fat and protein.

Simple, but not necessarily easy. I had to relinquish the carb/fat and carb/protein combinations that I had come to reply on. My beloved potato with butter and wild salmon became a potato with a big salad, and I ate the salmon separately with avocado and olives.

I love this formula, because it works for stabilizing blood sugar without having to give up carbohydrates. I tend to respond better to positives and additions than to negatives or limitations. Wrapping my carbs in fiber has been easier on my digestion, too. This is what I call a gentle approach to food discretion and managing blood sugar!

Of course, I always feel best when I choose non-starchy carbs, pay attention to how foods combine in my belly, and stay mindful of portions.

PRACTICE #7: MOVE YOUR BODY DAILY (FIND THE JOY!)

Move frequently at a slow pace.

—Mark Sisson

Moving your body is mandatory for getting healthy and sustaining wellness. It's simply not an option to not move; you are not meant to be sedentary. You need to move your body to strengthen your immune system and muscles, reduce inflammation, transport glucose from your blood to your cells, support deep sleep, maintain a steady mood, burn stored fat, and much more.

However, if moving your body is not fun and enjoyable, there is a high probability you will not continue the activities you start. That's just the way it is for most of us.

Contrary to popular belief, this is good news, and here's why:

Rather than focusing on pushing forward full steam ahead and dreading the next moment of exercise, you can take a gentler approach, and allow the art of practicing to support you in discovering a refreshingly uplifting life.

In fact, Dr. Chris Kresser says we should "move like our ancestors." They weren't running marathons or monitoring themselves with heart gear. They weren't swimming repetitive laps for 45 minutes or practicing power weight lifting. They performed low-intensity movements, such as walking and gathering food, accented by short periods of higher-intensity movements, such as hunting and fighting for survival. They were extremely fit, and the modern diseases we know of today were relatively absent.[32]

Think outside of the box. Let yourself dream to discover, and don't judge or edit. Just go.

Ask yourself, "What activity can I look forward to that will support me in moving my body in a fun and enjoyable way?" Here are some ideas:

- Walk in your neighborhood while listening to music or podcasts.
- Clean or organize your home vigorously while listening to your favorite music.
- Dance for 30 minutes every day in a dark room with candles and music.
- Splash around in a pool, river, or ocean; pretend you're a dolphin.
- Discover (or rediscover) the freedom and joy of bike riding.
- Jump wildly on a rebounder (mini-trampoline) for lymphatic massage.
- Get into nature and move intuitively to your heart's content.
- Take a dance, yoga, or Pilates class; experience your spirit rising.
- Find a friend who wants or needs to move too; move together.

NOW FOR A BIT OF PHYSIOLOGY

When you eat carbohydrates, they are converted to sugar in your bloodstream. This signals your pancreas to release the hormone insulin. Insulin sweeps in to take the sugar and move it from your blood to your cells. This is a natural process that allows you to receive cellular energy, giving you the ability to function and do whatever you need to do.

With type 2 diabetes, pre-diabetes, metabolic syndrome, or even before diagnoses or any symptoms arise, your carbohydrate-sugar-pancreas-insulin-cell process may not be working efficiently. If enough sugar is not moved from your blood and allowed into your cells, you will experience high blood sugar. This can result in unwanted health conditions over time, and low or intermittently low bouts of energy.

Let's clear the playing field … and here's where moving your body comes into play.

In an ideal world, insulin effectively moves the sugar from your blood to your cells. This may not be the case for you if insulin resistance is at play, but there is something else that will help move the sugar from your blood to your cells without the help of insulin: movement.

Regardless of how inefficiently your insulin/cell relationship is working, moving your body will help transport the sugar from your blood to your cells. This is why it's unquestionably effective to move your body after eating a meal, especially a heavy meal. If you feel sluggish or weighed down, get out and walk for 15 to 20 minutes. You will feel relieved.

If you experience insulin resistance, take notice. Moving your body helps get sugar out of your blood and into your cells. To some degree, it puts you on the same playing field as your (non-insulin-resistant) friends. Remember this:

Moving your body moves the sugar.[33]

Dr. Joseph Mercola says, "Inactivity is the primary risk factor for inactivity is the primary risk factor for insulin resistance."[34] If that doesn't get you moving, I don't know what will. After I read that, I definitely upped my game on moving my body.

FIND THE JOY

A necessary key to moving your body daily is discovering the joy in the practice. Whatever type of movement you choose, infusing it with playful anticipation and delight will make moving your body easier. Experiment to find what suits you best, and refrain from comparing yourself to others. Everybody is at a different place on the body-movement continuum; do what is unique to your character, fitness level, and joy meter.

There is no exercise you *should* be doing other than the one that brings you joy. Get creative, and make it happen. Walk while listening to music, a podcast, or an audio book; you'll be amazed at how quickly time seems to pass. Turn up your favorite songs and dance yourself silly in the comfort of your home. Splash like a child discovering water for the first time in a nearby lake, ocean, river, reservoir, or pool.

Keep it simple, and accept moving your body as a mandatory activity every day.

You are not alone if you need support in this area. Walk with a friend or family member, join a walking or hiking group in your community, work out at a gym or YMCA, or move and groove to a yoga or dance DVD at home.

No excuses: get moving.

ON A PERSONAL NOTE

It was 2009 in Oakland, CA, when I ditched my car, a small blue Mazda, appropriately named *Boy Blue*. I had been a solo car owner and driver for close to three decades. Having spent most of that time in bustling, traffic-heavy Los Angeles and Alameda Counties, three decades felt more like five.

Various circumstances merged into a stressful intersection of my life that led me to rid myself of the hunk of metal and become car-free. This was such a blessing! My partner and I walked the streets and avenues of Oakland and Berkeley, chanting our mantra: "Walking it off and walking it in; we're walking it off and walking it in." What we were walking off and walking in wasn't altogether known, but it didn't matter. We felt amazing.

Sooner than expected, over a short number of weeks, we went from walking two or three city blocks feeling arduous to walking two or three miles feeling like a breeze. It was exhilarating and in-spiring. We knew we were healing a myriad of issues across the board—physically, emotionally, and spiritually.

Day and night we walked. Errands, groceries, movies, and late-night events, we walked. From that point, walking became a life-long practice in managing my blood sugar, tapping into and releas-ing emotions, and expanding my joy-factor.

On my morning hikes, I walk with intention. That's to say, walking is part of my morning ritual (Practice #8). It's holistic in the sense that I actively engage my body, mind, and spirit as I move step by step for 30 to 50 minutes, up and down slightly rocky trails.

Throughout my walk, as I actively engage my spirit by paying attention to the world around me and to my breath, I convene with glorious nature. Spiritual practice is *here*. Spirituality lives inside of me, and nature is a great reminder of the present moment.

Big nature—oceans, mountains, rivers, forests, and trees—puts my so-called "problems" into perspective. The depth of the beauty and aliveness pulls me out of my own limited ego-reality mind and helps connect me to oneness—empty, full, quiet, present vibration.

***

My relationship with moving my body changed when I discovered that I loved to listen to podcasts while walking through my hilly neighborhood. I began noticing the flowers and variety of trees, interesting clusters of people, and patterns in house architecture and luscious gardens. I discovered a new sense of freedom.

I was so fully engaged and inspired (I love to learn) while listening to podcasts that 50 minutes passed with little effort, and before I knew it, it was time to head home. I entered into a mind-quieting practice of gratitude, affirmation, visualization, and forgiveness. I forgave myself for any judgments I had made against others or myself.

As I write about nature and spirit, I wonder if there is a familiarity that resonates with you—or if it feels esoteric and distant from your reality. Everything cannot be expressed in practical terms, and I believe this is one of those things. The value comes from the experience. It's definitely not an intellectual idea; it can't be blueprinted from reading words—digitally or in print.

It is when I embody the experience, and literally breathe it in, that my spirit opens and elevates me to new heights.

PRACTICE #8: CREATE A MORNING RITUAL (INCLUDE GRATITUDE)

> I choose to make the rest of my life the best of my life.
>
> —Louise Hay

It cannot be denied there is something magical and spiritual—awe-inspiring, breathtaking, and moving—in the morning. Before the shuffle and rumble of people, places, and things, there exists a tremendous opportunity to infuse your day, your life, with the qualities you desire. Is it peace you desire? Is restoration or calm on your want list? How about greater fulfillment in work, creativity, or income? Do you have needs in the relationship area?

Creating and sustaining a morning ritual sets the tone for your day and puts you in the driver's seat for creating a gateway to your life's vision.

Morning hours evoke a time of connection and devotion—to yourself, to the earth (literally the dirt that surrounds you), to your community, to the collective unconscious, and to the higher power of your beliefs.

Growth (inner and outer), personal empowerment, letting go of the past, becoming present, strengthening communication skills, expressing your art, excelling at work, increasing your revenue, and releasing disease … these things happen over time by way of daily practice, and the morning hour is where it all begins.

Why?

Personal growth begins in the morning when (and if) you are NOT starting your day responding to others. Take the opportunity to start each new day, a.k.a. your brand-new life, by paying attention and tending to the whole of who you are, your essence—body, mind, and spirit. Lean in without distraction, to anchor your full presence—the heartbeat of who you are. In a very real sense, you are messaging the universe—"I am here; I have arrived." Start your day with *thank you*.

The formula is not scientific, so I can't explain it in a scientific way. Rather, the explanation lives in the experience. It is different for everyone, of course, but I offer you a guarantee of self-expansion if you stick with it.

If you feel crazed, fast-paced, or jam-packed in the morning, you may find it challenging to consider morning hours as a necessary practice time. I simply ask you to start by devoting 15 minutes of your time. Here are some ideas for your morning practice: meditation, journaling, reading a blessing/positive-affirmation or inspiring book, visualizing what you desire, moving your body, drinking water with lemon, and reciting gratitude.

GRATITUDE

Actively engaging in a daily practice of gratitude is one of the most effective healing tools available. Gratitude is incredibly useful in transforming discomfort of all kinds, and in supporting the manifestations you desire. Like success, it feeds on itself and requires consistency and commitment. If you're already practicing gratitude, you know how powerful it is. If this is new to you, you will be delighted at how a mere five minutes of consistent daily practice can change your life.

Gratitude practice just works—period.

Close your eyes, open your heart, breathe deeply, and say "thank you" to whatever comes to mind in the moment. Don't overthink it. I often say, "Thank you for this breath. Thank you for the birds I hear right now outside my window. Thank you for time-freedom and flexibility. And thank you for my home in the mountains." Thank you goes a long, long....................way.

ON A PERSONAL NOTE

Daily morning ritual is my core practice. It's the first thing I do every day, and on the rare occasion I skip it, I miss it. I don't mean "miss it" in a light, breezy, oh-well sort of way. Rather, along the magnitude of not eating for a day; my footing and grounding are off. That said, I don't beat myself up about it; some days just go that way.

This is what my morning ritual practice looks like:

I generally wake up around 7:00 a.m., though this fluctuates. I plug in my iPod and choose *Chakra Mediation Music* by Stevin McNamara.

After brushing my teeth, I prepare a glass of room-temperature water with either fresh-squeezed lemon or a capful of apple cider vinegar. I hold my glass up to my kitchen window (often sighting deer eating blooms from the tree), say cheers, and begin to drink.

I nestle in my warm, comfortable meditation corner in front of large forest-facing windows. With the day before me, I sit on three propped pillows with a soft blanket by my side. My tools include an inspirational book, a journal, black and red pens for writing and underlining, a book light, and my glass of water on the window sill slightly above me.

I get comfortable, take some deep breaths, and say, "To the depth of my being more than anything else today, I choose to experience the love that I am." This is my mantra, a line from the book, *Coming Home* by Martia Nelson, which I read many moons ago.

My meditation practice is a combination of presence awareness (by quietly naming the sounds I hear to bring me back to center), affirmations, visualizations, and stretching. I raise my arms up high, breathe deeply, and make a circular movement to bring them back down. Clearly, a video would be more effective in describing what this looks like!

I end this part of the practice when I feel complete. It is an intuitive feeling (or sometimes just impatience) that may arise in 10, 15, or 20 minutes. I open my eyes and gaze out the window with a soft smile. It isn't forced or programmed; it's truly how I feel after meditating. After a few sips from my water glass, I move on.

This is the time I pick up a book. At the time of this writing, I am reading *A New Earth* by Eckhart Tolle for the second time. This time around, I find myself reading smaller sections in each sitting. I find sacredness in digesting just one message, then putting the book down. And yes, I underline passages … most definitely.

Journaling begins. I once heard someone call it "scribing"; I like that. Often, I'll write some notes about what I just read. Perhaps thoughts from yesterday, feelings that are present, or worries and concerns from mind-on-overdrive. Most of the time, my mind is not on overdrive first thing in the morning. This, of course, is one of the benefits of practicing upon rising.

Onward to an alkalizing, micronutrient-rich, life-enhancing veggie juice or green smoothie!

I grab my iPod and headphones and head out for my walk in big-nature. I listen to a health, writing, or business podcast, point myself in the direction of the hills, and walk up and down rocky trails for 30 to 50 minutes.

Upon returning home, I cool down and drink more water. If I

need to eat right away (which may be the case, post–green juice and workout), I eat.

Lastly, I open Scrivener (a writing software) on my computer, pull up uninterrupted meditation music on YouTube, and begin my writing session. I generally write 30–60 minutes daily, as I am doing right now.

PRACTICE #9: TAP INTO YOUR SPIRIT'S CALLING (EXPRESS, CREATE, & SHARE)

Make the most of yourself by fanning the tiny, inner sparks of possibility into flames of achievement.

—Golda Meir

I will do my best to emphasize how important this practice is.

You are meant to live BIG, not merely survive. If your creative juices are locked up due to daily obligations, or if you feel stuck in a rut with where your life seems to be, I guarantee 100% you can help move that energy to create the life you envision for yourself.

Finding what makes your heart sing and creating an outlet to express it isn't for just some people; it's for all people. Everyday people. In fact, it's your birthright and responsibility. You see, other people will heal from your wisdom, creativity, and insight. This is why the world is a fruitful and plentiful place.

Fulfilling your calling goes deeper, and here's how it connects to your health: if you're living as a machine, at the mercy of obligations and old routines that fail to serve your life force, you'll likely get caught somewhere between a high-stress rollercoaster and chronic addiction.

Creative self-expression is the missing ingredient to optimal health, a.k.a., a life well-lived. The story goes: as you create, you live; as you live, you create. Your purpose, second only to giving and receiving love, is to express, create, and share your gifts. Share with one person or a thousand; extend your hand.

If you do not know where to begin, start with a morning ritual practice! Just open this door, and your intuition will point your way forward. I know this to be true based on experiences from multiple people who continue to shape their lives by finding and trusting the calling of their heart's rhythm, me included.

The practice of creative self-expression does not need to be grandiose. In fact, it is the daily, incremental consistency that takes your seed of an idea and supports its growth into full manifestation. Much like building those model airplanes my father and younger brother whittled away at—one piece, a little glue, another piece, some more glue—small steps lead to big results.

Kris Carr, in her book *Crazy Sexy Cancer Tips*, says,

> Each of us has an inner reservoir, a deep well from which we draw healing waters. But when we stop paying attention or extend ourselves too far, we overlap the source and drain the magic juice. If your well is depleted, then it's time to fill 'er up.[35]

THE FALL

Visualize yourself on a teeter-totter, a grade school seesaw. Creative self-expression is the balance point in the middle; it's the queen pin between chronic stress-responses and addiction. Detouring too far from your spirit's calling (the center of the seesaw) may land you in habitual patterns of disease (hitting the ground on one end of the seesaw).

Dismissing your creative expression leaves you vulnerable to the fall. The fall is characterized by chronic stress and addiction. Why is this so? What is the bridge that leads to illness? It's made up of tiny bits and pieces of self-judgment, sometimes unrecognized because you think you're doing what you're *supposed* to be doing, regardless of your deeper intent.

Missing the mark here makes you a target to what lurks on either side of creative self-expression—chronic stress-responses and addiction. It's easy to miss your calling—sometimes, you only hear it through a quiet, subtle voice of guidance that echoes through your intuition. If tapping into your intuition and taking action based on what you sense is new territory for you, get still and listen.

Consider this stress-response syndrome: If you're moving through life mindlessly, plowing through from one heart-empty task to another, multiple subtle stress-responses may be triggering you in the course of just one day. The stress-responses present as self-judgment and judgment of others. You know those little criticisms that consistently arise as you continue to push through the "work" you desperately do not want to do? That is stress, and you pay the price for it.

The problem is that on the deepest level, your being knows it must create. Without creation, there is emptiness, the sorrowful notion that "I thought there was more to life." Inevitably, the self-judgments will come: Why am I at this job? I shouldn't be here; I'm worth more than this; I'm not living up to my full potential; I'm stuck; I hate it here (wherever here is); so-and-so is doing [fill in the blank]; I can't get ahead; if only …

Finally, however subtle, the moments of "I am unworthy; I am not good enough," creep into your psyche. This zone is fertile ground for chronic stress and addiction. Overexposure to stress-responses leaves you hovering in the shadow emotions—anger, envy, jealousy, frustration, detachment, and sadness—for too long. They become your way of life.

GET OFF THE ROLLERCOASTER

I am not suggesting that you can quit your nine-to-five job overnight, leave or transform a friendship that produces unending conflict, or not meet your familial obligations. I am also not suggesting the opposite.

What is important is getting the good stuff in. Just like with food, focus on bringing in more of what supports and nourishes you. The rest will fall away in due time.

Get your hands in the clay or in the garden. Write or draw to your heart's pursuit. Start that yoga class or take a hike in the woods. Begin that project you have always dreamed of, or dream it up now. Learn how to swim or teach someone how to dive. Embrace technology and social media or take a long-needed rest from it. The list is endless.

However, to do any of this, you must listen to your intuition and take action.

Living empty creates imbalance and breeds ill health because you'll need to reach for something to curb the pain, right? What will you grab? Food (either sugar or another drug) is fulfilling for about 15 minutes. It meets your immediate need, doesn't it? For such a drastically short period of time …

Food and other drugs will never meet your deeper needs—will never provide heart-centered connection to others, yourself, and the planet. Sugar and other drugs are *only* able to lead you into a downward spiral. Can you begin to see the critical need to express yourself creatively? Creativity is the center-point that prevents stress and addiction.

Bottom line: If you have a hobby, craft, or activity that brings you joy, do it. If it's been dormant due to some very good "reasons," push it up to the top of your list. Don't fool yourself into thinking you can't because of time; that's simply a story you have learned to recite. We all have stories we tell ourselves, most of which are half-truths. As the late author and poet Stephen Levine said, "The mind can be a useful tool but not a very good friend." YOU manipulate time; you are in the driver's seat. And if you aren't … you need to be.

I had a spiritual teacher, Wendy Spiller, who studied with Louise Hay. She said we could shrink or expand time. I have used this mind-bending tool effectively for decades. Now you can use it to create your art-life. Design it and sculpt it as you like. Move activities like musical chairs, cut out the pieces that no longer serve your highest good, and rearrange.

ON A PERSONAL NOTE

My creative self-expression is one of the most important aspects in my life. In fact, I separate "work" from "art." Work is when I'm freelancing for others—writing, editing, coaching, and managing projects. Art is connected to my life's calling—book-writing, content-development, teaching, training, and speaking.

During my daily walks, my first 20 minutes include mantra, gratitude, visualization, and prayer; this opens my day with creativity. I walk in wide-open spaces, often surrounded by big trees, blooms of all kinds, and, at times, a flowing creek that looks and sounds more like a river. In the early hours, people pass by in tidbits, unseen for the most part.

I move my hands and body to the vibration and rhythm of

whatever I'm expressing, often jiggling about. This allows me to release any sticky, mental loops that have seeped into the pores of my existence. Perhaps this makes up for moments in the day when I suppress expression—consciously or unconsciously holding back or simply choosing to refrain.

This embodied experience is the reason I rely on practicing to a large extent. It's a known element in my life with a familiar pathway: intentional, consistent action. The outcome may be drenched in mystery, but the path is not. This is the light I follow, and the glow that illuminates my way.

Once I recognized my calling—to teach, write, speak, and be a conduit for natural healing—I developed a fierceness to not let anything get in my way. Life has a way of presenting obstacles in the form of time, money, health, and other people's needs. My journey is a juggling act, for sure. Sometimes it feels like I'm fighting the good fight.

Coming to a deeper understanding of when I'm doing work vs. when I'm doing art has been significant. It's not that art time is all play and no work, or that working doesn't tickle my creativity. The difference is found in the intention, the purpose, and the calling.

PRACTICE #10: GET SUPPORT

Life is not a solo act. It's a huge collaboration, and we all need to assemble around us the people who care about us and support us in times of strife.

—Tim Gunn

Whether you are on a path to prevent or reverse type 2 diabetes, venture into healthy living, overcome food or other addiction, or simply want to feel better (physically or mentally), it takes a village—it takes team effort and support. We don't heal in isolation; we heal together in community. We heal as we commune.

When staring at your reflection in the mirror is not enough (and it rarely is), the right guidance from someone just ahead of you on the path can provide insight and increase your probability of transformation. For most people, getting well is not a solo endeavor. Support helps break the cycle of isolation and opens possibilities yet unseen.

After all, isolation is part of the collective mess that got us into this sick-cycle in the first place. Isolation is the type of fuel that puts distance between you and healthy living. Reclusion is a strong force that feeds on itself, creating a downward spiral. It allows too much time for your thinking mind to wallow in worry and distress and to snowball out of control. This level of stress can alter your body's functions and wreak havoc.[36]

Support whispers, "You belong." Community exists, even when you don't see it or realize it's missing from your life. It takes willingness to reach out and ask to connect—and, yes, it can be awkward. It's worth it, though, because support increases joy and reminds you that you are not alone in your struggle and daily practices.

Find support that works for your individual disposition. As in nutrition and health, there is no one-size-fits-all. The best time to reach out to a friend, mentor, coach, community group, counselor, class, or family member is now. Don't let money stand in your way either; support is available via paid or free services. Be willing to do a bit of research, and commit to the task of finding the support you need, in ministry to yourself.

ON A PERSONAL NOTE

Isolation has been detrimental to my physical and mental well-being. I was a quiet child and adolescent, philosophical and inwardly-focused. I did not feel understood or accepted by society or my community. I did not have a sense of belonging. Isolation breeds isolation, which wasn't good for my soul.

My mind found wide open spaces to run amuck, creating intricate maps laden with self-judgment and self-doubt. I was a go-it-alone person, and in many ways, I still am. While I am a self-proclaimed, proud introvert, introversion is not a mandatory sentence for isolation.

I've garnished support from therapists (the effective ones), 12-step meetings, friends, beloveds, books, online mentors, Meetup groups, YouTube videos, and family members; variety suits me. When I am open and ask for what I need, the right support comes at the perfect time.

I sense this is a lifelong practice for me—reaching for support, asking for help. Sometimes that knowing I need it is obscured, hidden by my weariness. Receiving support is a precious gift, and when it's first-rate, it's *wow*!

PRACTICE #11: LEARN YOUR SUPPLEMENTS

> Plant compounds have tremendous impact on our cellular functioning, but today we consume fewer plant micronutrients than our ancestors did, making supplementing our diet with vitamins, minerals, and other micronutrients a form of health insurance.
>
> —Dr. Steven Gundry

I'll start this chapter by reminding you to check with your health practitioner before changing or starting any nutritional supplement program or routine.

If you're taking chemical pharmaceuticals to lower your blood sugar, realize that effective supplementation will help to do the same. You may be able to lower or possibly discontinue pharmaceutical use altogether. Again, this should be navigated with your healthcare provider.

Nutritional supplements, including food-based vitamins, minerals, enzymes, and herbs, are *medicine*. They provide healing, and should be taken seriously. High-quality nutritional supplements can have profound positive effects on your blood sugar and provide protection against complications from type 2 diabetes.[37]

Everything has a context, and so do herbs and supplements. They are meant to supplement your nutrient-dense, anti-inflammatory, alkalizing, organic, whole-food, conscious-living lifestyle, NOT replace it. There is no miracle pill—natural or not—that will do for you what super-charged plants in their whole form will do.

> **You can't escape raising the bar on what you eat,**
> **drink, and how you live, and expect an herb or**
> **supplement to heal you.**

The absolute best way to consume vitamins, minerals, and enzymes is through whole, unprocessed food; make that your main course. However, with the rampant toxicity in our planet today—in all our systems, including food and water—it is imperative that you supplement your clean food plan and healthy lifestyle with effective, high-quality supplements.

HIGH-QUALITY ONLY

Nutritional supplements need to be high-quality, period. If they aren't, there's simply no point in taking them; you will be wasting your time, money, and health. You must find and choose companies that go the extra mile for your health, as their dedicated mission and value. Three companies I know I can rely on and trust are Mega-Food, Garden of Life, and Oregon's Wild Harvest.

Always read "other ingredients" first. This will save you time in choosing your supplements. If you see fillers or additives, which you will see most of the time, move on. It's silly, and I'll be blunt: ingesting un-pure, "dirty" supplements will do the reverse of helping to heal imbalance.

Look for fillers and additives such as magnesium stearate, vegetable stearate, soy lecithin, silica, dioxide, sugars, and dyes. The fillers are made so the manufacturer has an easier time moving the product through machinery without sticking; they are anti-glue agents. The additives are added to prolong shelf life and contribute to an attractive look and taste.

Brands with integrity, who produce high-quality supplements, find other ways to make it work. They search out "other ingredients" that are natural and harmless to create a product that is actually *health-based*. An example of a non-toxic ingredient that aids manufacturing but doesn't injure you is extra virgin olive oil. You will rarely see it because it costs more to use than magnesium stearate.

LET YOUR SUPPLEMENTS EVOLVE

It's important to realize that, as you change by implementing holistic lifestyle practices, your supplement regime will likely evolve. Drop the mindset that keeps you clinging to what once worked or what you read last year. Nothing is etched in stone. Your recovery will pivot back and forth in an unfolding progression; make room for adaptation.

You are your own best guide, which means you must learn to listen to your body and intuition, and make choices from that guidance. If this sounds abstract, or you're not sure how to tap in, start with Practice #8: Create a Morning Ritual. Your guidance will be revealed.

While I can't ethically tell you exactly what supplements to take, because this book is not individually tailored, when it comes to reversing or preventing type 2 diabetes, pre-diabetes, or metabolic syndrome, here is a list to carefully explore. I advise you to consult with your healthcare practitioner regarding:

- Cinnamon
- Alpha Lipoic Acid
- Gymnema Sylvestre
- Chromium Picolinate
- Magnesium
- Vitamin D
- Vitamin C
- Vitamin E
- Omega-3 Fatty Acids

The recommended dosages on bottle labels are usually maintenance dosages (for liability purposes) and not necessarily aligned with reversing disease. I'm going to share the suggested daily dosages of a handful of supplements that Dr. Julian Whitaker suggests for his diabetic patients, and you can take it from there.[38]

- Alpha Lipoic Acid: 200–600 mg
- Gymnema Sylvestre: 400 mg
- Chromium Picolinate: 400 mcg
- Magnesium: 1000 mg
- Vitamin D: 400 IU
- Vitamin C: 2000 mg
- Vitamin E: 800 IU
- Omega-3 Fatty Acids: 2–4 1000 mg capsules
- Bitter Melon: 2–4 oz
- Vanadyl Sulfate: 100 mg

ON A PERSONAL NOTE

I have fun with supplements—I really do. The artistic labels, high-integrity companies, and medicinal support add to my joy-factor. I love being a laser-focused investigator, mapping my way to the highest-quality supplements available. It's rewarding to establish connections with the products and brands.

My array of colorful bottles stands lined up on my kitchen counter, visible, not tucked away in a cabinet or drawer. And you know those handy-dandy pop-open containers labeled with each day of the week? The ritual of opening each supplement to lay out the week's supply keeps me organized and makes the process fun.

Finding pure, uncontaminated supplements is a continuous undertaking. While I am loyal to brands that keep their products free from additives and fillers, companies can change their tune. On more than one occasion, I've been surprised to see an additive, such as magnesium stearate, in a product that didn't have it on my prior purchase.

When this happens, I either withdraw from the company completely, or I continue taking its other products. It does make me wary, however, to continue with the company at all, because I can't help but question its integrity. Generally, I stay with brands that are 100% committed to the highest quality possible. If this means they need to dig deeper to find a great solution, they do.

One of the supplements I take is the antioxidant alpha lipoic acid (ALA). While ALA is well known for fighting free-radical damage and protecting cells, it is also fabulous in supporting healthy blood-sugar management. It aids in converting sugar to fuel, preventing the sugar from lingering endlessly in the bloodstream.

Try to find a clean alpha lipoid acid—I challenge you. Rummage through the shelves in your local grocer or health food store, and see what you find. I've searched many times to my dismay. Every bottle I've turned over was loaded with additives, oftentimes more than just one. It took me a long time, but I finally discovered an online supplier that made a pure ALA—SuperiorLabs, based in San Diego, CA. They went the extra mile for my health, and to that … I tip my hat.

PRACTICE #12: CHEW YOUR FOOD UNTIL LIQUID

> The more you consciously chew, the more con-
> nected you become to your food.
>
> —Jill Ettinger

It's the simple things, often overlooked, that prove to be most effective. Many daily practices, for instance, are free of charge and
accessible, without need for special tools or gadgets. Chewing your
food until liquid is a simple yet powerful practice.

Research shows that the state of your gut equals the state of
your health.[39] I cannot emphasize enough how important good digestion is to your overall health and quality of life. Digestive disor-
ders rank as our society's number one health complaint and top-of-
the-list reason for doctors' visits.

Chewing your food until liquid breaks down large particles of
food into small particles, making it easier to digest. You do not
want large particles of improperly chewed food to remain undigest-
ed in your intestines, collecting bacteria, putrefying, and creating
digestive problems.

On *The Model Health Show* podcast, Dr. Jillian Teta explained that the mechanical process of breaking down food, which starts with chewing, is hugely important. The crushing and grinding action of your teeth begins to predigest food, which reduces the stress on your stomach as the mechanical and biomechanical digestion process continues.

Dr. Teta emphasized the importance of allowing the digestive enzymes in your saliva to do their job, which primarily is to start the breakdown of carbohydrates. Chewing your food well will help to prevent the discomfort of gas and bloating, and reduce the risk of your gut bacteria highly fermenting the food.[40]

Another benefit to chewing your food until liquid is that it gives you a greater capacity to absorb the nutrients from the food. When you consider food as it relates to your health, it's not merely about what you eat; it's about what you absorb. If you're not absorbing the vitamins, minerals, and enzymes of the food you eat, you're not reaping the nutritional benefits.[41]

Chewing your food until liquid takes practice. Do the best you can. If you can't quite manage liquid, just break it down as much as possible. This practice will slow down mealtime. You will become present with the experience of eating food—its tastes and textures, along with the realization that you are eating in the first place.

The repetition as you chew will create sensation in your jaw; you may even get tired. You'll likely begin to notice others who are racing through their meal in a state of unconsciousness, and it might feel absurd to you. This is progress. Just keep chewing. …

ON A PERSONAL NOTE

A few years ago, when I was living in Santa Cruz, CA, I did an experiment. I set the intention and committed to chewing my food until liquid for 30 days. It turned out to be a practice I genuinely enjoyed.

The first thing I noticed was the extent it slowed down my eating experience, while, at the same time, raising my awareness of eating altogether. I remember sitting at the kitchen table, looking out the window to the backyard. With each chew, time seemed to extend, and I noticed myself becoming still and focused.

Chewing my food until liquid was significantly different than "a few chews and down the ole gullet," as I have done on many occasions. As I chewed, I sat. As I chewed, I noticed myself chewing. As I chewed, I became present to the current moment.

It's difficult to express the benefits of meeting the present moment; it sounds esoteric at best. It's one of those things that until I got there, until I was actually having the experience, the rewards seemed distant, unexplainable.

In fact, I would say it is a Zen-like, meditative experience. I believe any practice that slows me down and heightens my awareness of the moment has to be a valuable, life-affirming tool. Slowing down my eating helps me feel at peace, no rush, and no place to be but *here*. I recognize that many effective holistic health practices are simple in nature.

This 30-day experiment was a practice of mindfulness—eating mindfully, fully conscious, and undistracted. There was joy; I remember feeling joyfully content. Sadly, when I rush forward or drop awareness, the way I eat is different from those 30 days. It's simply a matter of a practice falling behind.

This is what practices do; they dip and swerve, glide in and seep out. Then, like a flip of a switch, awareness emerges, a new decision is made, and we are wedded to our practices again.

PRACTICE #13: PRACTICE STRESS-REDUCTION DAILY

> The greatest discovery of any generation is that
> human beings can alter their lives by altering
> the attitudes of their minds.
>
> —Dr. Albert Schweitzer

The link between stress and disease has become obvious to us as a culture. What was once considered abstract or arcane in regard to stress-related illness is now understood as fact. High stress is unquestionably linked to insulin resistance and type 2 diabetes.[42] In any case, it doesn't take a scientist or scientific research to inform you what the effects of stress feel like.

While symptoms are different for everyone, common symptoms of high stress are heartrate acceleration, sweating, a feeling of loss of control, exhaustion, and jumbled digestion. At a time when stress is at an all-time high and part of everyday life, concern over symptoms like these may be too easily minimized.

During the stress response, a physiological inside view would show your adrenal glands working hard, releasing the hormone cortisol. Your blood pressure and blood sugar rising, and your entire physiological ecosystem disrupted. Why take this lightly? It may be normal, but it isn't *good*.

STRESS ARISES

Stress arises from multiple places, including our environment, food-like products, relationship conflict, work and study deadlines, oppression, technology frustrations, care taking of a loved one, personal worries, ill health, death, birth, lack of funds, and abundance of funds.

What's tricky about stress is its indescribable nature. When you "feel stressed," what exactly does that mean? It shows up differently for everyone and doesn't feel good. This is because your immune and nervous systems are being attacked, causing metabolic chaos.[43]

THE STRESS-RESPONSE

Stress is not about stress; stress is not even about stressors—those bumps in the road life throws at you just because. With regularity, stressors arise, and they will continue to visit you during your duration on Earth. This we know; this we can't change. You *can* seek to minimize stressors by making significant changes in areas of your life where overstimulation occurs. These areas may include work; relationships with friends, family, and peers; housing; time management; and, of course, your health.

While removing stressors is possible, it is not an end-all solution, because the causes of stress are often out of your control. Since most of us can't escape stressors altogether, it's imperative to practice how we respond to those stressors through stress-reduction. Practicing stress-reduction techniques daily will train your body/mind/spirit system to respond to stressors intentionally in a way that supports your health and doesn't take control over your well-being.

If stress is not about stress or even stressors, what is it about? **The impact of stress on your mental and physical health boils down to your stress-response.** This, my friend, IS in your control … or it can be, with practice.

When you fall into a stress-response, your adrenal glands release cortisol. This causes your blood sugar to rise and creates an inflammatory response. If this only occurs occasionally, you don't have a problem. However, if you experience multiple stress-responses in a day or week, your adrenal glands will eventually become overworked and burnt out. This can lead to adrenal fatigue—a condition that is exasperating and takes a great deal of time and energy to reverse.

On top of adrenal fatigue, excessive stress means your pancreas is working overtime, trying to keep up with the demand for insulin to move the glucose into your cells. This creates a yo-yo effect between your adrenal glands and pancreas that gets worse and worse. Sadly, the *normal* inflammation response never has a chance to come back into balance. You develop chronic inflammation that inevitably leads to disease.

Stress overload alters your immune and nervous systems and wreaks havoc on your cellular function. It is as critical to manage as what you put in your mouth. Dr. Gabriel Cousens, author of *There Is a Cure for Diabetes*, writes, "Extreme stress for months at a time has been known to trigger the onset of a diabetic physiology."[44]

STRESS-REDUCTION PRACTICES

Stress-reduction isn't found in a pill, potion, or supplement. While there are herbs called nervines that have a calming effect on your nervous system and relieve mild anxiety—such as valerian, skullcap, kava kava, passionflower, and California poppy[45]—these should be used as an addition, not a substitute, for stress-reduction practices.

Being at the mercy of ongoing stress responses puts you at risk for physical and psychological symptoms. These symptoms hinder your quality of life and may lead you headfirst into type 2 diabetes and other conditions, including obesity, gastrointestinal problems, cardiovascular disease, fertility problems, immune suppression, depression, and thyroid problems.

Daily stress reduction practices (don't wait until the stressor arrives!) such as meditating, walking in nature, listening to music, cuddling with an animal or human, deep breathing, yoga, and resting, will create spaciousness as you respond to unpleasant situations.

Practice is the key to creating and sustaining greater calm and presence to meet life's stressors gracefully. Don't wait to begin your practices until the stressor arises; that is not effective. Begin today and commit to a daily practice. The practices can slide into your morning ritual beautifully.

Experiment: find what works for you and begin. Softening your stress-responses will allow you to be present in your life—the key to everlasting joy, vitality, and plenty.

Stress-reduction can be practiced in a variety of ways. Here are some ideas:

- Walking or sitting meditation
- Immersing yourself in nature
- Deep breathing
- Gentle physical activity
- Yoga or Pilates
- Guided visualization
- Rest / sleep
- Listening to soothing music
- Taking a hot, bubbly bath

- Enjoying a cup of organic herbal tea
- Losing yourself in your art

ON A PERSONAL NOTE

For the first three decades of my life, I didn't get angry very often. From time to time, sure, but nothing big-tempered or persistent. Then I hit my forties, graduate school, and the unpleasant symptoms of type 2 diabetes—mood swings, body shakes, rashes on both sides of my body, and emotional irritation.

Hello, anger.

It was as if anger was stored up in a tiny bottle, and when there was finally no more room to move, it blew. Yelling, stomping, throwing eucalyptus branches at doors …

It wouldn't be until many years later that I realized I needed to have a daily stress-reduction practice to soften my responses when triggers arose. Are my responses perfect now? Hardly. However, there has been much progress. Mere moments of pause or slowing down between stressor and response can make a world of difference.

How do I practice?

I meditate most mornings for 10 to 20 minutes. When my mind drifts, I begin naming the sounds I hear—birds singing, radio upstairs, house creaking, water pump swirling, chakra music playing. This brings me back to a center-point of presence.

I practice visualizations, affirmations, and gratitude at various times throughout the day.

I walk in big nature; some might call it a hike. I integrate hills and switchbacks—up and down, up and down. This centers me, helps move the sugar (inevitably, there is sugar from carbohydrates) from my blood to my cells, and produces a state of calm as my parasympathetic nervous system awakens.

I also take leisurely, intentionally slow walks (no hills except the ones I can't avoid, as I live on a hillside).

I gaze out my windows into big nature.

I burn natural, pure (remember, no chemicals) incense and *palo santo*—wood from a mystical tree that grows on the coast of South America. The aromatherapy is calming.

I rest as often as possible, listen to music, and watch videos.

I say no to *more* … more and more.

I take tasks and events off my plate, cancel and reschedule appointments and meetings, and clear my calendar when I start to feel overwhelmed or overstimulated. In truth, I often don't do this soon enough, and the overwhelm has crept in and wedged itself deeply into my psyche.

I cuddle, hug, and hold my beloved—healing, comforting, and affirming. This is body language doing what it does best: restoring goodness, allowing me to let go.

Ah yes … I take many hot baths, including bubbles when I remember to purchase the small herbal-infused packages.

I read, read, read. Always learning.

I cry.

I rejoice.

I give thanks.

I remember who I am. *I am.*

PRACTICE #14: INCREASE RAW PLANT FOODS (INCLUDE LEAFY GREENS, SPROUTS, & VEGGIE JUICE)

> A lot of people ask me what the best time of day to juice is. My answer: whatever time works for you, tootsie!
>
> —Kris Carr

Using plants for food, and better yet, as medicine, will provide you with generous benefits. Increasing your raw plant-based foods, while eating animal-based proteins in moderate proportions, sets into motion the transition from an acid-based internal ecosystem to an alkaline one.

This transition is significant to your health because acidity creates inflammation and alkalinity reduces inflammation. Inflammation is a known cause of many illnesses, including heart disease, diabetes, and cancer.[46]

Plants are loaded with micronutrients—vitamins, minerals, and enzymes. Cooking begins to destroy critical micronutrients, which is good reason to increase your intake of raw, living vegetables, fruits, nuts, and seeds.

Raw nuts and seeds are your friends. Devour the deliciousness and please do not worry or focus on the fat content. On the contrary, the monounsaturated fats found in almonds, pecans, macadamia nuts, and Brazil nuts, have been shown to improve insulin sensitivity.[47]

Leafy greens are among the highest *superb medicine*. They are loaded with an array of vitamins, minerals, enzymes, and antioxidants. These antioxidants fight free-radical damage, which helps to prevent cancer. Eating a variety of leafy greens is key to getting as many of these powerhouse goodies as possible. It's important not to cook them dead, as a significant portion of the vital nutrients will be lost that way. You don't need to eat 100% raw; 5 to 7 cups a day will do just fine.

Here is a short list of leafy greens to consider integrating into your daily meal plan: spinach, kale, dandelion greens, chard, and romaine. Include medicinal herbs such as parsley, arugula, and cilantro.

SPROUTS

Sprouts, such as broccoli, alfalfa, and mung bean, contain loads of plant protein and fiber, powerful antioxidants, and support cell regeneration. From sunlight to plant to animal …

If you think cow-food (beef) has a lot of protein, consider what healthy cows eat: grass. Every plant food started with a sprout and grew from there, and plants are loaded with nutrients. These powerhouse babies contain iron, magnesium, phosphorus, potassium, manganese, riboflavin, copper, protein, thiamin, niacin, vitamin B6, pantothenic acid, fiber, and vitamins C, K, and A.

Sprouts contain concentrated nutrients, which puts them in a class all their own. From the wisdom of Dr. Joseph Mercola: "The vitamin E content, for example (which boosts your immune system and protects cells from free radical damage) can be as high as 7.5 mg in a cup of broccoli sprouts compared to 1.5 mg in the same amount of raw or cooked broccoli. The selenium content can go from 28 mg versus 1.5 on the same scale."[48]

One of the greatest benefits of consuming sprouts is their enzyme factor. They contain proteolytic enzymes that make carbohydrates and protein digestible. While your body does produce enzymes, the process begins to wane over time, from a lack of consuming enough enzyme-rich, plant-based foods. Do yourself a favor: load up on whole food, plant-based enzymes, including sprouts. Let digestive enzyme supplements be a secondary support, as all supplements should be.

VEGGIE JUICING

Veggie juicing has been a medicinal and spiritual practice for centuries. When you extract the pulp and consume the liquid, you get a straight shot of powerful plant micronutrients (phytonutrients) into your blood and cells. This creates immediate detoxification, nutrition, and healing.

The plant matter is broken down and predigested for you (in the juicer); therefore, digesting takes little effort and has minimal impact on your organs. Your entire digestive system gets a chance to rest, restore, and repair.

One of the most potent and effective ways I know to reverse type 2 diabetes (and other conditions) is to juice organic leafy greens, vegetables, roots, and herbs. This creates nothing short of total transformation, and is not a new theory, fad, or diet; juicing is a centuries-old health and healing practice.

Veggie juicing is one of the quickest ways to create an alkaline system and transform an overly acidic body. As mentioned above, acid creates inflammation; inflammation and toxicity are known causes of disease. The idea is to move from an acidic meal plan and lifestyle to an alkaline one. At the root of juicing is the act of cleansing and detoxification. You must remove the old sludge that has built up over time and accumulated in your colon and intestines.

Acidic foods include most animal products, processed and junk foods, pharmaceuticals, sugar, coffee, sodas, and some plant foods. An acidic lifestyle is one ridden with constant stressors matched by unhealthy stress-responses. Yes, an overload of stress met without calm presence is acidic.

Blending is not juicing unless you pour the blended liquid through a mesh bag or strainer. Understand, the idea is to remove the fiber (pulp) in order to give your system a rest from the energy it takes to digest. The energy can then be used for your body's own healing process.

JUICING FRUIT

In the case of blood sugar control, to prevent and reverse pre-diabetes and type 2 diabetes, juice mainly vegetables, leafy greens, herbs, and non-sweet fruit such as cucumbers and tomatoes. While you might notice people consuming fresh juices with loads of apples, carrots, and beets, this is not recommended if you are pre-diabetic, diabetic, insulin-resistant, have high blood sugar, or experience metabolic syndrome. This is why I refer to the practice of juicing as "veggie juicing," and not simply "juicing."

Shawn Stevenson—author, nutrition expert, and co-host of *The Model Health Show*—spoke about lipogenesis, a process where fructose (fruit sugar) mainlines straight to your liver. He called it a "fat production factory," where triglycerides (fat in the blood) are produced. This leads to insulin resistance (the foundation for pre-diabetes and type 2 diabetes), inflammation, and fat storage in the belly. There is no question why we are seeing astounding rates of non-alcoholic fatty liver disease in children: their consumption of soda pop containing high fructose corn syrup is out of control.[49]

JUICING APPROACH

Rather than approaching juicing as a fast, I suggest integrating veggie juicing into your regular food plan. This is different than doing a juice fast or juice feast, which would require deeper introspection into your current level of wellness and disease, and would be best monitored by a holistic healthcare practitioner.

Veggie juicing is powerful medicine. Because you are removing the fiber (for medicinal purposes), the nutrients will move into your cells and blood at astounding speed. Your blood sugar will rise, as it does with anything you eat or drink. As insulin comes in to move the sugar to your cells, your blood sugar will drop. You need to gauge your own response to the rise and drop of your sugar and energy level. You may need to eat a light meal 30–60 minutes before and/or after drinking your juice.

Incorporate 8 to 16 ounces of fresh, organic veggie juice into your daily food plan. Start with a base of celery and cucumber. Add leafy greens (kale, spinach, collards, romaine, chard, or dandelion). You can add ¼ apple or ½ to 1 carrot for sweetness if you need to. Other options include lemon, ginger, turmeric, parsley, and cilantro.

There are lots of questions when it comes to juicing, e.g. "Which is better—juicing or blending?" "What kind of juicer should I use?" "How much and how often should I juice?" "Where are the juicing recipes?" Because juicing is a book in itself, and not the sole focus of this book, I have created a free eBook as a supplement. "5 Medicinal Green Juice Recipes & Easy Start Guide."[*]

---

[*] http://drnickisteinberger.com/waveresources

Have fun juicing; it is a unique and enriching experience!

In addition to eating fruits and veggies in their whole state, or juicing and blending, Matt Monarch, author of *Raw Success*, has created the largest online raw food and superfood store in the world. The Raw Food World[*] is my go-to store for the highest quality raw foods and superfoods on the planet.

ON A PERSONAL NOTE

The raw foods movement is a lifestyle, and it changed my life in 2010. It spoke to me right away; I felt intrigued and lured.

I remember finding Dan McDonald, "Dan the Man," the *Life Regenerator*, on YouTube. He had a juicing table and juicer setup in the great outdoors, in front of his RV camper. His spark of vibrant health touched a chord in me, as I watched him cut veggies and fruit and feed them through the chute of the juicer.

Years later at a farmer's market I frequented in Oakland, CA, I saw Dan sitting off to the side, in a patch of grass and rocks. He was talking to a group of people about raw foods. I moved in closer to listen, super excited to be in the energy. Out loud, I thanked him for the impact his teachings had had on me. I shared that I reversed type 2 diabetes holistically. He reached into his green canvas bag, pulled out one of his DVDs, said "Congrats," and tossed it my way.

From the start of my reversing-diabetes journey, I began eating lots of raw plant food: veggies, leafy greens, fruit, nuts and seeds, and gourmet raw meals and desserts. Green smoothies loaded with superfoods and veggie juices were part of my daily menu. I ate about 75% raw foods, and, for two years, plant-based only.

There's something unquestionably enlivening about eating raw

---

[*] http://drnickisteinberger.com/rawfoodworld

plant food, and it has to do with the magnificent array of living enzymes. I wasn't used to feeling elated after eating. Just the opposite; I'd spent years feeling heavy, tired, and weighed down. This was definitely a new and engaging experience.

I had many "aha" moments that propelled me to quickly join the juicing club. Without question, my intuition-based knowingness kicked in. I felt on the mark, fun, and captivated. I loved the creative aspect of putting a new mix of ingredients together. Cooking has never been my strong suit. Spices, timing, and temperature never came naturally to me. In fact, it was a common occurrence that half the food I cooked stuck to the bottom of the pan.

Preparing raw food was a different experience altogether. I got the gist of it quite quickly, and it made logical sense to me. Salads, smoothies, juices, nut milks, and raw cereals ... no problem. The kitchen became my friend. I started playing around with raw cacao (chocolate that is naturally low in sugar and super-high in antioxidants), lucuma powder (low-glycemic sweetener, rich in nutrients, derived from the lucuma tree in South America), blended nut milks (including almond, cashew, Brazil, and hemp seeds), chia seed porridge, and loads of new vegetables and leafy greens.

PRACTICE #15: GET GOOD SLEEP

> A good laugh and a long sleep are the two best cures for anything.
>
> —Shawn Stevenson

Sleep (or lack of it) affects everything you do ... everything. It can make or break your mood, tax or elevate your energy level, decrease or increase blood sugar, support insulin resistance or sensitivity, and help you store fat or release it.

Sleep deprivation and too many nights of ongoing low-quality sleep will compromise your immune system and become a catalyst for conditions such as obesity, diabetes, depression, memory loss, and cancer.[50]

It's not only the quantity of sleep you get, although that's important, and studies show that most folks need a good eight hours optimally. The quality of your sleep is just as important as how much you get—perhaps more. Strive for deep, uninterrupted sleep with good air ventilation in a dark environment.

If you take sleeping pills (a.k.a. chemical pharmaceuticals) to help you sleep, you probably know you are among many who have found relief with a pill. You also may be one of many who have become addicted to these power-hitters, and perhaps you are curious if there is another way.

Here's where lifestyle practices come in ... and patience. If you want to kick the habit, you must gradually layer effective lifestyle practices that will help you sleep more deeply. While it's not an overnight process (no pun intended), you can get there with natural methods.

Herbs are hard-hitters too, generally with positive side-effects. Maybe you've tried some herbs that haven't worked for you. It's about finding the right combination for your particular make-up. Consider blends of valerian, California poppy, kava root, passion-flower, chamomile, and skullcap. Magnesium in the later hours is wonderful too. Often when taking herbs, it is not one plant that does the trick, but a combination of a few or many. As always, check with your healthcare provider before making changes to your medical or healthcare program.

Remove EMFs (electromagnetic frequencies) from the room where you sleep (wi-fi-generated devices especially); disconnect and unplug all power sources, especially cordless phones and wi-fi routers. Get off your computer, phone, or tablet and stop eating at least two hours before bedtime. Keeping these devices on will keep you buzzing away through the night. Do not underestimate the power of these radioactive monsters (spoken by a big techie with multiple devices).

There's something that folks often miss, or haven't been educated on: sleeping with all natural linens—100% organic cotton, hemp, bamboo, and wool. This goes for any sleep clothes you might wear as well. Synthetic (poly) fibers are toxic endocrine disrupters[51] that can and will disrupt your sleep.

One of the biggest toxic giants you own is your mattress. This is what you breathe in all night long. If you have access, replace your mattress with an organic cotton/wool/latex (natural rubber) mattress. Do your research to find the least-toxic mattress that fits your budget.

ON A PERSONAL NOTE

If you are one of those people who sleep deeply night after night with no significant issues, deem yourself fortunate. Insulin swings, hormones post-50, a creatively aggressive entrepreneurial mind, and failed supportive mattress attempts have left me sleep-deprived on many nights.

In 2016, my year of midlife-crisis awakening, I wrote a fun and meaningful blog post about my experience. For approximately nine months, I traveled through parts of Southern and Northern California, and Southern Oregon. I shacked up with friends; stayed on couches and back porches; cared for houses, dogs, cats, and fish; and slept many nights on my portable camping cot.

The thing about the camping cot (frame: Coleman, bed: REI) is I slept really well. I'm not sure why a $200 twin size (arms tucked into blankets, so they don't hang off the bed) outdoor mattress and foldable metal camp cot had me sleeping better, deeper, and more peacefully than my newly purchased socially acceptable mattress set. At any rate, the camp cot lives long and dies hard. It's in my back room, so when I need to trade off from my conventional bed, I use it.

Oh, mattresses—soft, firm, in the middle. Too soft, too firm; need a topper. Toxic, less toxic, 100% natural, expensive. I don't want those nasty chemical and glue endocrine disrupters. What to do …

I did my best with a less toxic mattress and a cotton-plus-synthetic mattress topper. I had to return the down-filled topper because the feathers were poking through into my skin. Somehow, bird feathers in the bed just didn't sit right.

Managing blood sugar when insulin resistance is at play does not allow me to sleep through the night— any night—without getting up to pee two, maybe three, times.

I sleep best in cool or even cold weather. I would say it's the post-50 women's hormone scenario, but my younger brother is the same way. I need fresh air, no matter what the temperature is outside. Thirty degrees—give it to me. It wouldn't be the first time I froze out a beloved or family member, or was told I created an arctic zone.

No breath, no life.

Sleep on.

PRACTICE #16: RELEASE
PROCESSED FOODS

Observe yourself and your behavior without judgment. Positive feelings and compassion make it easier to make a better choice next time.

—Mary Toscano

Processed foods—or, rather, food-like products—are dangerous, and a root cause of disease.[52] Filled with chemicals; processed sugars; iodized salt; and rancid, oxidized oils, these products are highly addictive and alluring. If you're anything like me, you may struggle with keeping your distance from these unnatural items.

They're convenient, aren't they? Pleasantly wrapped or boxed with colors and verbiage that seems to speak directly to you. This is the case until your taste buds change and say *yuck*. This is the case until you change from a gradual process that arises from practicing.

You may have associations from childhood or other areas of your life that keep these cravings top of mind. Know that it's not all in your head, however; not simply a matter of willpower. Once those powerful substances enter your body, they create an addictive response.[53] In fact, according to Dr. Mark Hyman, "Sugar and processed foods have been shown to be eight times more addictive than cocaine."[54]

Your body does not know what to do with these food-like products, but it has learned to adapt.[55] Too bad you don't have a mirror or bionic vision to your organs, cells, and blood!

Speaking of blood, diagnostics that detail your blood work can be helpful in giving you a peek inside. If your LDL (low density lipids) cholesterol is high, turn down the processed foods and watch it shrink.

The typical Western meal plan is loaded with processed foods. I quoted it earlier, but it's worth quoting again. According to Dr. Steven Gundry, author of *Dr. Gundry's Diet Evolution* and *The Plant Paradox*: "When a primitive culture adopts a Western diet, and particularly refined carbohydrates, within one generation its people begin to experience the typical diseases of the civilized world. Hypertension, diabetes, heart disease, arthritis, cancer, and colitis— diseases currently unknown or rare in such cultures—become rampant."[56]

Be gentle with yourself; don't beat yourself up. Always seek to upgrade the quality of ingredients in the food and drinks you're consuming. Transitioning to eating only whole, healthy foods affects many of us on a deep emotional level. As you ride the highs and lows of your journey, simply make the best choices you can each day, and surrender when your choices don't meet your wishes and expectations.

At a certain point, processed foods will no longer be the highlight of your day. Not only will your body say NO, but your mind and spirit will also. You'll want something better for yourself, higher-quality because you are high-quality. It will happen; it's a process.

Go slow.

ON A PERSONAL NOTE

Regardless of what I know about health, healing, and illness—oblivious to my research and experience helping others and myself heal and prevent disease—processed foods still seem appealing. It's hard for me to believe, but it's true. If I wrote it any other way, I wouldn't be honest.

While I typically hold to a self-standard for consuming higher-quality ingredients in the sweet and salty realm—products without additives, chemicals, preservatives, and inflammatory oils, such as canola—at times I turn a blind eye.

My first reach is for lower-glycemic, healthier sweeteners, including coconut sugar, lucuma, mesquite, and fruit. Unfortunately, sometimes sweet treats made with these ingredients can be difficult to find. When I do find these sweeteners in baked goods, they often come with a longer list of other less appealing ingredients, like of tapioca starch, agave syrup, and canola oil.

There are times, places, and circumstances when I grab a Twix candy bar. I just do. (Perhaps when you're reading this, that won't be a reality anymore. I can hope!) When the want is real, the want is now. Conscious or unconscious, I rip apart the sparkling colored wrapper. ...

I don't beat myself up about it, by the way. What's done is done. It's a quick bit of instant gratification and pleasure. Honestly, sometimes it's not even enjoyable, particularly if I eat it fast or in a secretive way. The health nut can't possibly be seen choking down a highly processed, sugar-laden candy bar! Nonetheless, it's true.

Sugar is evil; it really is. It gets in and creates a Krazy Glue stronghold on my system—body, mind, and spirit. Perhaps you can relate? The thing is, I've come into acceptance, and stopped the fight. Does this mean I consume processed foods nonstop without repose? No. I rest, go long periods without the culprit, and make wise choices often.

In fact, ... I live a kickass life!

PART FOUR:
PRACTICE TO LIVE;
LIVE TO PRACTICE

RECLAIM JOY, VITALITY, AND PLENTY

Do you believe that joy, vitality, and plenty are your birthright? I do. I don't mean from an entitled or privileged position, but from the home of your spirit—the place where all is well if you get out of your own way.

We do get in our way, you know. It's really no fault of our own, as we are inundated with the pitfalls of negative messages and self-judgments that stem from big-media advertising, and funnel down into our communities and homes. How dare the outside world of big business try to tell you who you are and who you *should* be! How dare they?!

Joy, vitality, and plenty are what this ride is all about. Joy, vitality, and plenty build up defenses against illnesses, and squeeze them out until they have nowhere to exist. Remember, type 2 diabetes is a condition that lives in a particular environment; when you change the environment, you change the condition.

Preventing and/or reversing diabetes (or any imbalance) is a side note (a big one!) that happens organically as your system corrects itself over time.

How does the *Holistic Practices Lifestyle* tie in with reclaiming joy, vitality, and plenty? As you emerge and rise up (and you will), and as your daily habits and choices become more conscious, your natural inclination toward your own profound wisdom will move you forward. This becomes the breeding ground for living at your fullest potential, your deepest capacity.

Let's examine joy, vitality, and plenty individually.

JOY = PRESENCE

Joy can only be found in the present moment. I'm talking about deep, penetrating, everlasting joy, not the kind of joy that is fleeting, or riding the waves of external circumstances. Not the kind of joy you experience because you are happy as a result of liking something, or from experiencing instant pleasure. That kind of joy can never be everlasting because you will feel discontent when the bounty of your liking is not there. What I'm suggesting is the possibility of *permanent joy*.

Permanent joy is always present as long as you are present. By "present," I mean aware and conscious in the current moment. This phenomenon happens as you shift course from ego-identification (where you identify with form, things, situations, and circumstances primarily) and move toward identification with a deeper sense of knowing who you really are.

You may readily find your true nature by immersing yourself in nature, listening to music, meditating, walking, and other such mind-quieting, spirit-opening moments. You may also find your center in the 16 practices. When you raise your awareness, you raise your awareness. As you take steps to lift yourself to feeling outright amazing, a deeper sense of joy and contentment is the natural outcome. You don't have to trust me; practice and experience it for yourself.

VITALITY = ENERGY

Energy waxes and wanes, and most of us wish we had more. You may associate your energy level with your sleep cycle, age, health, or the activities of your day. It's hard to accept feeling wiped out or lacking vibrancy. Feeling tired midday or upon rising can trigger feelings of depression and self-loathing. Have you considered this: that your energy level may be impacted by your mindset, as well as the ebb and flow of your creative self-expression?

Food affects mood; food affects your energy level.[57] So does moving your body, sitting for prolonged periods, forgetting to affirm what you are grateful for, and being depleted of adequate micronutrients—vitamins, minerals, and enzymes. What you put in your belly and what you keep in your mind deeply impact your vitality.

As you practice daily, you'll notice your energy level improve. You'll get choosy about what and when you need to practice to balance or raise your energy. As you nourish yourself, your energy stores release to provide you with what you need. Holistic practices seek to elevate you, not bog you down. So rise up to the sun and celebrate to greet a new day of living.

PLENTY = ENOUGH

Not barely enough or just enough. Enough! Enough of whatever it is you need to fulfill the level of contentment that's in synergy with your inner world—that place of stillness where joy resides. Regarding *plenty*: there is a meeting of inner world and outer world, where we consider form, circumstance, and stuff.

When your experience of joy and vitality starts to hike up, you'll automatically feel more grateful and plentiful. If I make it sound like everything meshes or pushes into the next concept, that's because it does when you live holistically—in awareness of your body-mind-spirit connection. It's all connected.

I could apologize for not making it more scientific, but I won't. I'd rather you feel it than analyze it.

What do you need to feel full, whole, and complete? I encourage you to make a list. Then, surrounded by nature, in meditation, reflect on your items-for-fulfillment. You may get an insightful chuckle or a gem of wisdom. As you engage in the practices, notice how your list changes. See what you cross off and behold what you manifest.

AREAS SCREAMING OUT FOR MORE

When I work with clients in my holistic health coaching practice, I ask them to set an intention to open their eyes to the "areas screaming out for more." The 16 practices highlighted in this book cover a wide gamut of lifestyle areas. For sure—and this is true for everyone—your strengths and limitations will become obvious. Areas where you have practiced in the past will feel familiar and perhaps easy. New practices may feel daunting in the beginning.

I am guessing that you have excelled in certain areas, while others have trailed behind. If you take a detailed inventory of your body, mind, and spirit—what you've been through, what you've rejected, and where you've taken action—you'll notice where your attention has focused. As a teacher and holistic health educator, I encourage you to stretch into *other* areas … the areas screaming out for more. Draw your energy toward these places. By all means, continue doing what comes naturally, but also notice where you are being *called to attend*. If you're not sure how to discover this, an effective place to start is in Practice #2: Meditate a Minimum of 10 Minutes Every Day.

When I am asked which practices to start with, I guide folks in the direction of where their *pull* is. It's quite simple: if meditation comes easily to you, but walking feels like one hundred burdens, it's time to lace up and get walking. If you love to move your body and do it as daily ritual, but the idea of a big, bountiful salad every day just bums you out, it's time to hit your local natural grocer or farmer's market and get connected to the produce.

You must listen to your intuition for guidance, as it will always lead you to where you need to be. For the third and final time, I'll repeat the late poet and author Stephen Levine: "The mind can be a useful tool but not a very good friend."

Heed your calling.

YOUR WELLNESS JOURNEY CONTINUES

I hope you have found value in this book and feel ready to take your next unique step toward preventing and reversing type 2 diabetes (and other conditions) and reclaiming joy, vitality, and plenty!

If this transition feels overwhelming, I understand. Just know that taking action won't be difficult with proper support. Remember, this is not meant to be a solo effort. Teamwork is a key ingredient of success for all of us.

RESOURCES PAGE:

Here is where you'll find supplemental companion guides to use as checklists and a handy support system as you move through the practices. The book is ending, but practicing is a lifelong adventure and worthy commitment. The below guides are available on my resources page:[*]

- 10 Top Foods to Stock Your Kitchen for Optimal Health
- 7 Nutritional Supplements to Reverse Type 2 Diabetes
- 10 Holistic Lifestyle Practices to Prevent & Reverse Disease (beginning and advanced)
- 5 Medicinal Green Juice Recipes & Easy Start Guide (eBook)

Private Facebook Group: If you haven't yet joined us, swing by and see what's going on. This is a wonderful group of heart-centered people on their journey to wellness, just like you. Come get your questions answered and learn what practices are working for other folks. Joy, Vitality, & Plenty Community.[†] See you on the *inside*!

YOUR REVIEW OF THE BOOK

Thanks so much for reading to the end! I wholeheartedly thank you for your time and focus. To spread the word on the healing potential of these holistic practices, and to help folks determine if this book is the right fit for their healing journey, I would greatly appreciate your honest review.[‡]

Wishing You Joy, Vitality, & Plenty!
xo Dr. Nicki

---

[*] http://drnickisteinberger.com/waveresources/
[†] http://drnickisteinberger.com/community
[‡] http://drnickisteinberger.com/wavereview

NOTES

[1] Ganda, O. P. (2018). Diabetes and heart disease – an intimate connection. Retrieved from http://www.joslin.org/info/diabetes_and_heart_disease_an_intimate_connection.html

[2] Carr, K. (2015). Crazy sexy juice: 100+ simple juice, smoothie & nut milk recipes to supercharge your health (p. 20). Carlsbad, CA: Hay House Inc.

[3] American Society for Metabolic and Bariatric Surgery. (2013, November). Type 2 diabetes and obesity: Twin epidemics. Retrieved from http://asmbs.org/resources/weight-and-type-2-diabetes-after-bariatric-surgery-fact-sheet

[4] Cousens, G. (2008). There is a cure for diabetes: The tree of life 21-day+ program (p. 6). North Atlantic Books.

[5] Hyman, M. (2016). Eat fat, get thin: Why the fat we eat is the key to sustained weight loss and vibrant health (p. 189). New York: Little, Brown and Company.

[6] Grimm, J. J. (1999). Interaction of physical activity and diet: Implications for insulin-glucose dynamics. Public Health Nutrition, 2(3A), 363–8. https://doi.org/10.1017/S136898009900049X

[7] Menke, A., Muntner, P., Batuman, V., Silbergeld, E. K., Guallar, E. (2006). Blood lead below 0.48 micromol/L (10 microg/dL) and mortality among US adults. Circulation, 114(13), 1388–94. https://doi.org/10.1161/CIRCULATIONAHA.106.628321

[8] Healogics. (2016, November 1). Healogics treating chronic diabetic wounds with advanced therapies. Retrieved from http://www.healogics.com/11-01-16-PR-Diabetes-Awareness

[9] Cleave, T. L. (1974). The Saccharine Disease. Bristol, UK: John Wright & Sons.

[10] Gundry, S. R. (2009). Dr. Gundry's diet evolution: Turn off the genes that are killing you—and your waistline—and drop the weight for good (p. 18). New York: Crown Publishers.

[11] National Institute of Environmental Health Sciences. (2018, May 21). Endocrine disruptors. Retrieved from https://www.niehs.nih.gov/health/topics/agents/endocrine/index.cfm

[12] Schauss, M. (2015, June 30). Toxicity and chronic illness. Retrieved from https://www.westonaprice.org/health-topics/environmental-toxins/toxicity-and-chronic-illness/

[13] Zion Market Research (2017, January 11). Global dietary supplements market will reach USD 220.3 billion in 2022: Zion Market Research. GlobeNewswire. Retrieved from https://globenewswire.com/news-release/2017/01/11/905073/0/en/Global-Dietary-Supplements-Market-will-reach-USD-220-3-Billion-in-2022-Zion-Market-Research.html

[14] Joseph. (2016, August 24). Why anti-fat is completely misguided (and the mess it put us in). [Blog post]. Retrieved from https://lifeforbusypeople.com/2016/08/24/why-anti-fat-is-completely-misguided/

[15] Gundry, S. R., & Ehrman, W. J. (2005). Raising HDL with diet and supplements: Accomplishing the impossible! Diabetes and Vascular Research Journal, 3(2), 134.

[16] Jiang, R., Manson, J. E., Stampfer, M. J., Liu, S., Willst, W. C., & Hu, F. B. (2002). Nut and peanut butter consumption and rise of type 2 diabetes in women. JAMA, 288(20), 2554–60. doi:10.1001/jama.288.20.2554

[17] Hyman, M. (2016). Eat fat, get thin: Why the fat we eat is the key to sustained weight loss and vibrant health (p. 157). New York: Little, Brown and Company.

[18] Hyman, M. (2016). Eat fat, get thin: Why the fat we eat is the key to sustained weight loss and vibrant health (p. 27). New York: Little, Brown and Company.

[19] Davis, W. (2011). Wheat belly: Lose the wheat, lose the weight, and find your path back to health. Emmaus, PA: Rodale Books.

[20] American College of Preventive Medicine. (n.d.). Lifestyle Medicine Initiative. Retrieved from https://www.acpm.org/page/LifestyleMedicine?

[21] Hyman, M. (2016). Eat fat, get thin: Why the fat we eat is the key to sustained weight loss and vibrant health (p. 193). New York: Little, Brown and Company.

[22] Wilson, D. (2015, January 8). How inflammation and pain affect your sleep. [Blog post]. Retrieved from https://doctordoni.com/2015/01/how-inflammation-and-pain-affect-your-sleep/

[23] Tolle, E. (2005). A new earth: Awakening to your life's purpose. New York: Penguin.

[24] Earl, N. (2016). Relaxation 101 – How to activate the parasympathetic nervous system. Retrieved from http://healthvibed.com/relaxation-101-how-to-activate-the-pns/

[25] Hyman, M. (2016). Eat fat, get thin: Why the fat we eat is the key to sustained weight loss and vibrant health (p. 14). New York: Little, Brown and Company.

[26] Hyman, M. (2016). Eat fat, get thin: Why the fat we eat is the key to sustained weight loss and vibrant health (p. 80). New York: Little, Brown and Company.

[27] Simopoulos, A. (2002). The importance of the ratio of omega-6/omega-3 essential fatty acids. Biomedicine & Pharmacotherapy, 56(8), 365–79. https://doi.org/10.1016/S0753-3322(02)00253-6

[28] Gundry, S. R. (2009). Dr. Gundry's diet evolution: Turn off the genes that are killing you—and your waistline—and drop the weight for good (pp. 39, 108). New York: Crown Publishers.

[29] Gundry, S. R. (2009). Dr. Gundry's diet evolution: Turn off the genes that are killing you—and your waistline—and drop the weight for good (pp. 38–39). New York: Crown Publishers.

[30] Philip, J. (2011, February 26). Low fat diet missing essential brain nutrients and leads to cognitive decline. Natural News. Retrieved from http://www.naturalnews.com/031504_low-fat_diet_brain_function.html

[31] Toscano, M. (2013). Sweet fire: Sugar, diabetes, & your health (p. 35). Mary Toscano Healthy Living.

[32] Kresser, C. (2011, March 10). 9 steps to perfect health – #7: Move like your ancestors. [Blog post]. Retrieved from https://chriskresser.com/9-steps-to-perfect-health-7-move-like-your-ancestors/

[33] American Diabetes Association. (2017, September 25). Blood glucose and exercise. Retrieved from http://www.diabetes.org/food-and-fitness/fitness/get-started-safely/blood-glucose-control-and-exercise.html

[34] Mercola. (2017, April 21). Stand up, sit less, move more – especially if you are diabetic. Retrieved from http://fitness.mercola.com/sites/fitness/archive/2017/04/21/exercise-benefits-for-diabetics.aspx

[35] Carr, K. (2007). Crazy sexy cancer tips (p. 74). Guilford, CT: Skirt!

[36] Mercola. (2010, May 15). The physical toll of loneliness. Retrieved from https://articles.mercola.com/sites/articles/archive/2010/05/15/the-physical-toll-of-loneliness.aspx

[37] Whitaker, J. (2001). Reversing Diabetes (p. 161). Grand Central Publishing.

[38] Whitaker, J. (2001). Reversing Diabetes (pp. 203–205). Grand Central Publishing.

[39] Kresser, C. (2011, February 24). 9 steps to perfect health – #5: Heal your gut. [Blog post]. Retrieved from https://chriskresser.com/9-steps-to-perfect-health-5-heal-your-gut/

[40] Stevenson, S. (2016). TMHS 132: Digestion 101: Natural solutions for digestive health – with guest Dr. Jillian Teta. The Model Health Show. Podcast retrieved from https://theshawnstevensonmodel.com/jillian-teta/

[41] Boutenko, V. (2005). Green for life (pp. 62–65). Raw Family Publishing.

[42] Brandi, L. S., Santoro, D., Natali, A., Altomonte, F., Baldi, S., Franscerra, S., & Ferrannini, E. (1993). Insulin resistance of stress: Sites and mechanisms. Clinical Science, 85(5), 525–35. doi:10.1042/cs0850525

[43] Cousens, G. (2008). There is a cure for diabetes: The tree of life 21-day+ program (p. 56). North Atlantic Books.

[44] Cousens, G. (2008). There is a cure for diabetes: The tree of life 21-day+ program (p. 56). North Atlantic Books.

[45] Sinadinos, C. (2009). Stress relief with nervine herbs. Retrieved from https://www.starwest-botanicals.com/content/stress_relief.html

[46] Hyman, M. (2016). Eat fat, get thin: Why the fat we eat is the key to sustained weight loss and vibrant health (p. 96). New York: Little, Brown and Company.

[47] Rivellese, A. A. (2003). Quality of dietary fatty acids, insulin sensitivity and type 2 diabetes. Biomedicine & Pharmacotherapy, 57(2), 84–7. https://doi.org/10.1016/S0753-3322(03)00003-9

[48] Mercola. (n.d.). What are sprouts good for? Retrieved from https://foodfacts.mercola.com/sprouts.html

[49] Stevenson, S. (2014). TMHS 068: Boost your fat loss with these 5 tips for a healthy liver. The Model Health Show. Podcast retrieved from https://theshawnstevensonmodel.com/tips-for-a-healthy-liver/

[50] Stevenson, S. (2013). Sleep problems? Here's 21 tips to get the best sleep ever. Retrieved from https://theshawnstevensonmodel.com/sleep-problems-tips/

[51] Upaya Naturals. (2014, January 29). Toxic clothing – Dr. Brian and Dr. Anna Maria Clement. Retrieved from https://upayanaturals.wordpress.com/2014/01/29/toxic-clothing-dr-brian-and-dr-anna-maria-clement/

[52] Anand, S. S., Hawkes, C., de Souza, R. J., Mente, A., Dehghan, M., Nugent, R., . . . Popkin, B. M. (2015). Food consumption and its impact on cardiovascular disease: Importance of solutions focused on the globalized food system: A report from the workshop convened by the World Heart Federation. Journal of the American College of Cardiology, 66(14), 1590–1614. https://doi.org/10.1016/j.jacc.2015.07.050

[53] Schulte, E. M., Avena, N. M., Gearhardt, A. N. (2015). Which foods may be addictive? The roles of processing, fat content, and glycemic load. PLoS One, 10(2), e0117959. doi:10.1371/journal.pone.0117959

[54] Hyman, M. (2016). Eat fat, get thin: Why the fat we eat is the key to sustained weight loss and vibrant health (p. 190). New York: Little, Brown and Company.

[55] Allison, D. B. (2014). Liquid calories, energy compensation, and weight: What we know and what we still need to learn. The British Journal of Nutrition, 111(3), 384–86. doi:10.1017/S0007114513003309

[56] Gundry, S. R. (2009). Dr. Gundry's diet evolution: Turn off the genes that are killing you—and your waistline—and drop the weight for good (p. 18). New York: Crown Publishers.

[57] Aubrey, A. (2014, July 14). Food-mood connection: How you eat can amp up or tamp down stress. NPR. Retrieved from https://www.npr.org/sections/thesalt/2014/07/14/329529110/food-mood-connection-how-you-eat-can-amp-up-or-tamp-down-stress

Made in the USA
Columbia, SC
01 August 2020